LAUGH, CRY, EAT SOME PIE

LAUGH, CRY, EAT SOME PIE

A Down-to-Earth Recipe for Living Mindfully
(Even When the World Feels Half-Baked)

DEANNA DAVIS, PhD

A PERIGEE BOOK

A PERIGEE BOOK
Published by the Penguin Group
Penguin Group (USA) Inc.
375 Hudson Street, New York, New York 10014, USA
Penguin Group (Canada), 90 Eglinton Avenue East, Suite 700, Toronto, Ontario M4P 2Y3,
Canada (a division of Pearson Penguin Canada Inc.)
Penguin Books Ltd., 80 Strand, London WC2R 0RL, England
Penguin Group Ireland, 25 St. Stephen's Green, Dublin 2, Ireland
(a division of Penguin Books Ltd.)
Penguin Group (Australia), 250 Camberwell Road, Camberwell, Victoria 3124, Australia
(a division of Pearson Australia Group Pty. Ltd.)
Penguin Books India Pvt. Ltd., 11 Community Centre, Panchsheel Park,
New Delhi—110 017, India
Penguin Group (NZ), 67 Apollo Drive, Rosedale, North Shore 0632, New Zealand
(a division of Pearson New Zealand Ltd.)
Penguin Books (South Africa) (Pty.) Ltd., 24 Sturdee Avenue, Rosebank, Johannesburg 2196,
South Africa

Penguin Books Ltd., Registered Offices: 80 Strand, London WC2R 0RL, England

While the author has made every effort to provide accurate telephone numbers and Internet addresses at the time of publication, neither the publisher nor the author assumes any responsibility for errors, or for changes that occur after publication. Further, the publisher does not have any control over and does not assume any responsibility for author or third-party websites or their content.

Copyright © 2010 by Deanna Davis, PhD
Text design by Kristin del Rosario

First edition: August 2010

Library of Congress Cataloging-in-Publication Data

Davis, Deanna.
    Laugh, cry, eat some pie : a down-to-earth recipe for living mindfully (even when the world feels half-baked) / Deanna Davis.
       p.   cm.
    "A Perigee book."
    ISBN 978-0-399-53594-9
    1. Self-actualization (Psychology)   2. Consciousness.   3. Life.   I. Title.
    BF637.S4D375   2010
    158—dc22   2010005848

PRINTED IN THE UNITED STATES OF AMERICA

10   9   8   7   6   5   4   3   2   1

The recipes contained in this book are to be followed exactly as written. The publisher is not responsible for your specific health or allergy needs that may require medical supervision. The publisher is not responsible for any adverse reactions to the recipes contained in this book.

Most Perigee books are available at special quantity discounts for bulk purchases for sales promotions, premiums, fund-raising, or educational use. Special books, or book excerpts, can also be created to fit specific needs. For details, write: Special Markets, Penguin Group (USA) Inc., 375 Hudson Street, New York, New York 10014.

For my sisters, Kristie, Michelle, Alicia, and Verlie—you have always been (and always will be) my favorite people to laugh with, my safest people to cry with, and my most beloved fellow pie-indulgers.

And in memory of both Gary Holum and Renee Klosterman Power. Dad, thank you for teaching me how to savor both pie and life . . . what a gift you gave me! And Renee, your life was an unrivaled example of mindfulness and warmth . . . thank you, my friend.

ACKNOWLEDGMENTS

Here we go! A heartfelt thank-you to all of my audience members from the *Womanhood: The Divine Comedy* show, whose laughter and feedback helped refine these stories and the messages they carry. To all of the nonprofit organizations I have partnered with to bring this show to your communities and causes—the work you do is extraordinarily important and it has been a privilege to work with all of you! Special thanks to Transitions of Spokane for being the first organization to work with us, and to RiteCare Spokane for taking the concept to a whole new level.

Thank you, too, to my readers, clients, and event attendees—your desire to live life by design rather than by default consistently challenges me to learn more to better serve you.

Marian Lizzi, editor of my dreams, and Cathy Hemming, ever-faithful agent, you both rock my world! And to the wonderful team at Perigee, you make publishing not only possible but a real pleasure.

For your unconditional love and tireless support, which I never had to ask for, but which you always offered in the form of child care, emotional support, foodstuffs and beverages of various sorts, and practical contributions of all kinds to my life and business, I want to thank: Kristie, Dan, Brianna, Michelle, Mike, Jacob, Alicia, Blake, Verlie, Amber, Rhiannon, Chad, Malina, Carsten, Connie, Kay, Debbie, Kari, Susan, Lisa, Sara, Katie, Nicolle, Sue, Di, Rita,

Dianah T., Mark and Jim, Phyllis and Don, GG, and Karen. And to the Millers, the Klingbacks, and the Ehlerts—the world would be a better place if there were more friends and neighbors like you!

Julie Peterson, you and Renee shaped my life in more ways than you will ever know. Thank you both for supporting my personal growth and professional journey, for encouraging me every step of the way, and for your friendship. We all should be so lucky to have people like you stewarding our talents to serve the world.

Bob Maurer and Mary Anne Radmacher, you continue to enrich my journey as a writer and speaker, and I am honored to call you both mentors and friends. Brett Enlow, thank you for our many spirited conversations on mindfulness and what it really means.

Sally Pfeifer, you sparked my writing career during a chance conversation one day, and Peggy Herbert, you showed me the power of positive interactions to change people and the world. You are both examples of the transformative nature of education and the caring nature of human beings.

Michael, through all of it . . . and that's a lot . . . you are still my best friend and biggest fan. With you, every laugh is more luxurious, every tear is easier to bear, and every slice of pie tastes sweeter. I love you.

CONTENTS

Contents

CHAPTER 1

Why Pie

From Vice to Virtue

I didn't realize until tonight that I had chosen my career in large part so that I could not only *indulge in* and *validate* my many vices but also be *compensated* for sharing those vices and their requisite consequences with scores of people worldwide. This revelation happened when I sat down to write a blog post about my progress on the manuscript for the book you now hold in your hands. While introducing the title, since it deals with pie, something moved me to check the previous week's blog posts to make sure I wasn't fixating too heavily on one particular topic (such as foodstuffs, for instance). Yes, it's true that I have to run this little "checks and balances" system because I do, indeed, fixate too heavily on particular topics on a regular basis, which usually end up being related to one or more of my vices—most of which are food and beverage related.

So I scanned through those posts to find that I had begun the week by writing an exceptionally long piece (in blog years, where each paragraph equates to seven paragraphs due to our society's hopelessly short, Twitter-fied attention span) on "The Cheese-Free Me." This was an extended (but thankfully humorous) account of my decision to give up all dairy products on the recommendation of my chiropractor in an effort to reduce the inflammation related to my recent back injury. The piece detailed the trauma I experienced making the decision to go "cheese-free," and the subsequent expressions of both shock and horror it elicited from those who learned of my self-imposed fast. (It still seems, as I mentioned in *Living with Intention*, that cheese is one of the great unifiers of humankind.) I reviewed the next post, which described my latest chocolate escapades, followed by the post introducing this very book, which extols the life-affirming aspects of pie.

When I realized that at least half of that week's posts had not only *referenced* but actually *centered* on the topic of food, I had to make the editorial decision to postpone publishing my planned piece titled, "Fondue Haiku," in the event that my food fixation would undermine my credibility as a Positive Psychology and success expert (as if it hadn't already). Then I recalled the fact that, despite my expertise in the field, several advanced degrees, and my publishing credits, the only (and I mean *only*) element of my professional bio people recall after I give a keynote speech is that I "support the addition of chocolate as a key component of the USDA Food Pyramid."

So, after thinking about it for a while, I realized that I am, undeniably, blessed to be compensated for describing in detail the self-help strategies associated with my many vices. In my defense, I do my very best to frame aspects of those vices as virtues, since there are so many powerful lessons to be learned from the perfect slice of pie or a great pinot noir or a massive brick of creamy cheese. As such, I've informed my editor and wanted to let all of my readers know that from here on you can expect not only blog posts but also an entire book series on my various propensities for foods and beverages of various types. Yes, I'll share future musings on martinis, tomes on treats, paperbacks on pasta, writings on wine, and chapters on cookies. But for the purposes of this book, I'll narrow my focus to the strikingly significant benefits of pie.

The Late, Great "Cake or Pie?" Debate

There are cake people and there are pie people. I'm convinced that we're born with an innate preference for one or the other strategically embedded in our DNA to spur heated disputes about the correct dessert choice for Sunday dinners, summer barbecues, and family reunions. I also believe that this genetic programming extends far beyond the late, great "cake or pie?" debate to other questions of culinary choice such as coffee or tea, milk or dark chocolate, white or red wine, cookies or bars, vodka or gin, and cheese or, well, anything healthier (or less satisfying). These pairs at times unite us and at times polarize us. So just to get the whole unity/polarity thing off to a rip-roaring start, let me begin this book by stating that I am an unabashed and unapologetic coffee-drinking, dark chocolate–snacking, red wine–sipping, cookie-eating, vodka-swilling, cheese-nibbling *cake* eater.

This cake affinity is the reason why some people (including myself) find it a bit odd that I have just penned a book that not only extols the *virtues* of pie (rather than cake) but that also makes a compelling case for its use as an *instrument for self improvement*. To this latter point, I must say that as an equal opportunity foodie, I will selflessly promote the use of *any* fare that incorporates large quantities of either sugar or fat (ideally both) as a path to enlightenment. But if those were the only criteria for personal transformation, I would simply advocate bathing daily in Schokinag German drinking chocolate and be done with it. While I'd actually like to try that (I'll get back to you on my findings), I maintain that there are important, life-changing lessons to be learned from pie. Those lessons are simple: A great *pie* is all about what you put *into* it, and also about what you leave *out* of it. It's about the ingredients you choose, how you assemble them, how you respond to the unexpected, and the extent to which you savor both the *process* and the *product* of your work. And, as you've probably surmised, all of these things also apply to a great *life*.

> A great *pie* is all about what you put *into* it, and also about what you leave *out* of it. It's about the ingredients you choose, how you assemble them, how you respond to the unexpected, and the extent to which you savor both the *process* and the *product* of your work. And, as you've probably surmised, all of these things also apply to a great *life*.

With pie, there are certain ingredients that need to be included in the correct amounts to be sure you'll get the result you want (like sugar and spices). And then there are other ingredients less sensitive to the *amount* you add, since they're dependent on your personal *taste* (like apples and pecans). With most things you bake, some of the things that go into the recipe are appealing on their own (like berries and chocolate), some are sour but morph into something sweet (like lemons and rhubarb), and some are incomplete or unpalatable on their own but are absolutely standard in a rich, well-crafted pie (like but-ter and flour). And yet, when they all come together in that final, one-of-a-kind dish, mixed in the right proportions, effec-tively layered, exposed to just the right amount of heat, and allowed to gently cool, the result is a *pie* to remember.

The same recipe guidelines apply to life. There are certain things that need to be included in the correct amounts to be sure you'll get the results you want (like laughter and mindfulness). And, there are other ingredients less sensitive to the *amount* you add, since they're dependent on your personal *taste* (like con-nection and resilience). With most things in life, some of the things that go into the recipe are appealing on their own (friend-ship and fun), some are sour but can eventually morph into something sweet (like stressors and setbacks), and some are in-complete or unpalatable on their own but are absolutely stan-dard in a rich, well-crafted life (like tears and grief). And yet, when they all come together in that one-of-a-kind experi-ence, mixed in the right proportions, effectively layered, exposed to just the right amount of heat, and allowed to gently cool, the result is a *life* to remember.

Lest you are concerned that Julia Child will soon leap out of your pantry cupboard and start quoting Yoda or citing Tony Robbins, we can probably now move from the pie/life analogy into other pertinent topics. Such as why, as a lifelong *cake*-lover, I am a *pie*-baker-turned-pie-author, and why it even mat-ters, since if you're like most people, you're far more interested in your *own* life than you are in *mine*. We're getting there. Let's begin with, "Why pie?"

Why Pie?

The whole pie thing started when I was about twelve when, one weekend, out of sheer boredom and utter apathy, I started leafing through a 1950s James Beard cookbook that was buried underneath far less appetizing reads in my dad's library. In it, I found a simple apple pie recipe that I figured even *I* could pull off. I had nothing else to do and had all the ingredients on hand, and since there wasn't a single thing in my dad's house that would satisfy my colossal pre-teen sweet tooth (I'd already downed all of the humidity-damaged chocolate chips and had resorted to gnawing on chunks of hardened brown sugar to get my fix), I set out to bake my first pie as a simple, selfish act of desperation.

I pulled out the ingredients and got to work. I painstakingly followed the directions to make the pie crust, calling my grandmother repeatedly for phone coaching on the nuances of producing a flaky pastry. I peeled what felt like fourteen thousand apples with the most extraordinarily dull vegetable peeler to ever show its blade in a kitchen, until my hands cramped and beads of sweat rolled down my face. (Incidentally, this set the stage for my eventual codependent relationship with my Pampered Chef apple peeler/corer/slicer. Like my children, it has a named guardian in my will and will receive a portion of my estate in the event I meet with an untimely demise before it does.)

I carefully measured out the white and brown sugars, but stopped short when the recipe called for me to "dot" the pie with butter and "sprinkle" with cinnamon. What in the heck was *that* supposed to mean? How much constitutes a "dot," and exactly how does one measure a "sprinkle"? I was paralyzed for a few moments until I finally decided that I could either just give it my best guess or give up. The guess seemed more likely to produce a radical sugar high later in the day, so I opted for that option and proceeded to heap sweet, sticky slices of apples in layer upon layer, "dotted" with butter and "sprinkled" with cinnamon until the top crust strained and bulged as I sealed the edges.

I watched as it baked, all of the juices streaming over the sides and down into the bottom of the oven, eventually smoking my family members out of the house until the fire alarms stopped sounding. And then it was done. It was a work of art: perfectly browned, perfectly shaped, perfectly tender, and perfectly fabulous. As I took my first bite of my first pie, I felt entirely at peace (which I needn't tell you is not only *uncommon* but more accurately *unheard-of* in the altered reality that is the life of a moody, hormonal pre-teen girl). Though I didn't know it at the time, I was in a state of flow, of bliss, of culinary nirvana. And then, as I sat in silent reverie, modestly accepting the praise and adulation of my family members, it dawned on me: I don't even really *like* pie.

Yet I was beaming and I felt a rush of joy and contentment that proved to be a pretty sweet alternative (both literally and figuratively) to the daily practice of expressing my angst through dramatic and unfounded complaints about the injustices of life. Rather than medicating myself with risky behaviors and illicit substances, as many kids do, as strange as it sounds, I started to get high on pie. When the world seemed out to get me (and when *doesn't* it seem out to get a twelve-year-old?), I would take myself back to what it felt like to create that first model of pastry-wrapped perfection. I celebrated the patience and present-mindedness (not to mention the hard work) that it took, the mastery of a new skill, the ability to quickly respond to crises (like a smoke-detector symphony), the connection with others as they indulged in something I'd done to nurture and serve them (trust me, it didn't happen often), and finally the process of savoring the "fruits of my labor" in the form of the perfect pie. Pie as personal development. It had a ring to it.

Baking had suddenly and strangely become a form of self-discovery, self-expression, self-care, and even on occasion, self-sacrifice (particularly when I had to resort to using that damned vegetable peeler or when I had to offer the last piece of pie to an aged guest—curse decorum). It taught me that a good outcome is tied both to your preparation and to your flexibility, and that slight flaws don't ruin the finished product; in fact, those imperfections are unique signs that you lovingly handcrafted it. I found that, like in my apple pie, sometimes you don't even have to mix up the ingredients to produce what you want; instead it's the layers you add one by one that eventually meld together to create something exquisite. And, I learned that a good pie has to be exposed to extreme temperatures in order to turn out just right. I realized, years later, that all of these things were lessons for success both in pie baking and in life.

> I learned that a good outcome is tied both to your preparation and to your flexibility, and that slight flaws don't ruin the finished product; in fact, those imperfections are unique signs that you lovingly handcrafted it.

And then there's the whole practical rather than philosophical, and selfish rather than selfless side of the issue. When it comes to my apple pie, I've got to admit that honestly, I make that baby for *me* and *only* me. I really don't care if anyone else loves it or hates it (though what's not to love?), or even if anyone *eats* it, for that matter (except in the unlikely event they eat the last piece, in which case there's hell to pay or a limb to be lost). When I make that apple pie, it's all about *me*. So few things in life end up being just about *us*, so I milk this one for everything I can. While I bake it, I know *exactly* how fabulous it's going to be. I know what that first bite will taste like, and how luscious the after-dinner slice will be. I know precisely how amazing tomorrow's breakfast will be—a thick wedge, heated up and topped with a whopping slice of sharp Cheddar cheese and a steaming-hot cup of coffee. It's more than just a hedonistic act of self-care, though. Really. I appreciate that pie in advance. I savor it in the present. I express my gratitude for it after it's gone. I celebrate with it when things are going well, console myself with it when things aren't, and connect with others through its irresistible gravitational pull. In fact, I consider that apple pie to be the gift that keeps on giving in that it's an ongoing reminder that all of those things I just listed are just as important to my *life* as they are to my *pie*.

And Then There's the Whole Laughing and Crying Thing

As the title indicates, though, this book is about more than just the transformative nature of baked goods. There's the whole laugh/cry part of the recipe, too. Here's the link. In my many years as a speaker, author, and entertainer, I've had the privilege of working with thousands of people on the process of truly savoring their life experiences. And, I've searched for the best ways to help them adjust what they're putting *into* their lives in order to change their *outcomes*. In my books and presentations,

I explore all aspects of our life experience—the triumphs, the tragedies, and the absurdities (the stuff that you couldn't make up if you tried). And, I do my best to shine a light on the *options* you have to view different situations in your life in more productive ways and the *choices* you can make to influence those situations in meaningful ways. There is no "perfect recipe" for *designing* your ideal life, only your "preferred recipe" for *living* it.

> **T**here is no "perfect recipe" for *designing* your ideal life, only your "preferred recipe" for *living* it.

Without fail, as a speaker, the two comments I hear most often are, "I laughed until I cried," and, (just as powerful, if not more so), "I cried until I laughed." My audiences share how relieved they are to be invited (or reminded) to embrace a *range* of emotions in their lives, from sullenness to silliness and everywhere in between, and to purposefully decide *the meaning* they want to ascribe to each life experience. In fact, one of the common ingredients of a well-lived life is the ability to experience this array of emotions without being trapped by the assumption that you need to think or act a certain way in a certain situation. The choice is always solely and blessedly yours.

> **O**ne of the common ingredients of a well-lived life is the ability to experience this array of emotions without being trapped by the assumption that you need to think or act a certain way in a certain situation. The choice is always solely and blessedly yours.

Now, it's true that in these uncertain times people seem to be getting daily doses of either disappointment or devastation (sometimes both). We're faced with threats to everything from our financial health to our physical health and from global conflicts to global warming. Though people want more *satisfaction* and *success*, they often feel like they're experiencing more *setbacks* and *stress*. Rather than levity they feel anxiety, and peace gives way to panic. It's certainly enough to make you cry. "Thanks, Deanna," I can hear you say. "I feel *so* much better now. What would I have *done* if you hadn't so clearly articulated the many reasons for my current *despair*?" I promise we're not going to stay here. There's a point. Trust me.

We all know that challenges are a part of being human, and that they're just one ingredient in the recipe for life. *But we don't need to be defined by our disappointments*. Instead, we can make a conscious decision to learn what we're meant to from those experiences and choose to create something infinitely more palatable. It's the sum total of our experiences and our attitudes that make life both meaningful and memorable. That's why, even when a good cry is called for (and often it is), in most circumstances you can find *something* that provides a sense of relief if you commit to seeking it out. Indeed, it's often possible, even in the midst of hardship, to engage a fleeting smile, a tiny snicker, a welcome giggle, or (with luck) a full-fledged belly laugh.

> We don't need to be defined by our disappointments. Instead, we can make a conscious decision to learn what we're meant to from those experiences and choose to create something infinitely more palatable. It's the sum total of our experiences and our attitudes that make life both meaningful and memorable.

People understandably get so caught up in the drama of the day that they don't realize they have the power to reframe almost any situation (or at least a moment or two within that situation) into something more bearable simply by *changing how they look at it*. For me, that reframing usually comes in the form of laughter, an often unexpected but always welcome flood of lightheartedness that can help redefine a moment even in the darkest of times. And, if I can't muster laughter, at least I can turn to connection. Or mindfulness. Or release. Or distraction. And if all else fails (or even when all else succeeds) I can always resort to pie. Baking it. Eating it. Sharing it. And, as unbelievably corny as it sounds, *learning* from it.

That's what this book is about. Like pie, life is about artfully combining a variety of ingredients (some of which aren't all that pleasant on their own) and giving them a gentle stir to create something you can truly savor. It's about a dash of grace here and a sprinkle of humility there. It's also about leaving *out* what will spoil the flavor (like negativity and apathy) in favor of seasoning it to your liking with things like presence and purpose. It's about knowing that, in order to bake a truly great pie, you have to expose it to tremendous heat at some point to transform it into something unforgettable. Interestingly, the same holds true for human beings. Finally, it's about allowing it to cool—to rest—in order to enjoy it at its best. This is a recipe for living, an invitation to mix together the range of ingredients that life has to offer and truly savor the results. When in doubt, laugh, cry, eat some pie. And when called for, do all three.

The Recipe for Living Mindfully

Now, it's time for a quick overview of what you can expect from *Laugh, Cry, Eat Some Pie*. First, you'll find real-life stories on relationships and jobs (sometimes they're one in the same!), housework and stress (doesn't one *cause* the other?), and kids and crises (often synonymous) through topics like blue flip-flops and backup panties, speeding tickets and wandering weasels. They're also tales of friendship and food, love and loss, and humiliation and hope brought to you by the following sponsors: The Lasagna Fairy, Dr. Uptalker, former president Nixon, and none other than Chuck E. Cheese himself. Each story offers a laugh and a few may even summon a tear or two, but all contain im-

> Humor, it seems, alternately serves as a life *enhancer* and a life *preserver*.

portant lessons about life, laughter, and the pursuit of happiness. Humor, it seems, alternately serves as a life *enhancer* and a life *preserver*. And its accompanying tools for transformation include perspective, connection, adaptability, resilience, release, and mindfulness. Indeed, these are the ingredients for a life well-lived and we'll explore each in the following chapters.

Through these stories I invite you to engage in the present moment, regardless of whether it brings contentment, challenge, or sheer confusion. And, I encourage you to live more mindfully by simply immersing yourself in each experience and defining its meaning on your own terms. My favorite definition of mindfulness comes from Jon Kabat-Zinn, one of the leading experts in stress reduction and quality of life, who says that mindfulness is a matter of "paying attention, on purpose, in the present moment, nonjudgmentally, as if your life depended on it." My personal take on this definition is that it's about not only being *aware of* but also, and even more important, being *engaged in* what you are experiencing at any given moment, good or bad, pleasant or not, funny or sad.

Mindfulness is an invitation to live in the here and now with purpose and conviction and with a sense of lightness (and hope-fully lightheartedness!) rather than carting around all of your heavy baggage from the past or your weighty stack of fears and anxieties about the future. It's about being open to what you might learn both *about* and *from* yourself, others, and the world through your life journey. And, it's about how, when you are truly present and nonjudgmental about yourself and your expe-riences, you can make a deliberate decision at any time to change your *outlook* and thus your *outcomes*. Mindfulness allows you to consciously design your ideal life on your own terms in this moment, regardless of your external circumstances.

Indeed, Kabat-Zinn had it right when he concluded his def-inition of mindfulness with, "as if your life depended on it," though I want to share one important distinction. *Living* is a *process*; your *life* is the *product* of that process. Both are wor-thy of our attention and celebration. So, just as you must pay close attention to the *process* of baking in order to enjoy the *product* of a well-made *pie*, you must also attend to the *process* of *living* in order to enjoy the *product* of a well-lived *life*.

> Living is a *process*; your life is the *product* of that process. Both are worthy of our attention and celebration.

Now, to maintain this focus on mindfulness throughout the book, at the conclusion of each story you'll find a section called "A Slice of Insight," as well as one called "Mindfulness Bite by Bite." (Oh, come on. Nice try. You didn't *really* think I'd let you get away with a diet of only *entertainment* and *edibles*, did you? Alas, no, fair readers. A healthy mind—and life—requires the presence of the third "e"—*education*.) But, I've served it up on a silver pie plate for you. Your "Slice of Insight" is really just "food for thought," a summary of important concepts from each story. And "Mindfulness Bite by Bite" offers you three simple questions to help you enhance your *awareness* of important principles as they apply to your own life, and to help you take *action* in ways that will help you live the life of your dreams. Visit www.deannadavis.net to download your free copy of the e-workbook that includes handy worksheets for exploring your responses to these questions and your ideas for integrating what you learn into your life.

Finally, if you're like me—not that you'd necessarily *want* to be, as you'll learn from many of the stories contained in this book—but if you *are*, all this talk about pie has sparked a bit of an appetite for a little something of the pastry persuasion. If that's the case, you'll also find a few of my favorite pie recipes, along with their relationship to the topics at hand. For instance, you'll be introduced to the following recommendations: "When life gives you lemons, make lemon meringue," and "When faced with challenges, first sigh, then eat mud pie." With that, I think it's just about time to laugh, cry, and eat some pie. As a wise person once said, "Life is short . . . Eat dessert first!" Dessert is served!

CHAPTER 2

Perspective

What You Add to the Mix Matters

Strawberry-Rhubarb's Got the Power

One of the first pies that came to mind when I decided to write this book was the unbelievably, fabulously amazing strawberry-rhubarb pie made by White Box Pies in little old Spokane, Washington. Eating it can be a spiritual experience—it's that good. Or if a suggestion like that offends you, eating it can also be an entirely hedonistic experience that allows you to gladly direct your spiritual experiences elsewhere. Whatever works for you. One of the things that has always intrigued me about this variety of pie is that you can take something as spectacularly *foul-tasting* as rhubarb and pair it with something as universally *appealing* as a strawberries and, voilà! The result is nothing short of pure, unadulterated bliss.

In my opinion, the same holds true for life. Strawberry-rhubarb pie is a perfect example of how your *perspective* can impact your life. You can—and most certainly will—be faced with a wide array of unpleasant *inputs* in life, ranging from challenges and crises to disappointments and even devastation. But your *output*—your true quality of life and long-term contentment—depends exclusively on how you *mix* those experiences with other inputs and how you package them together to serve up generous slices of hope and happiness in life. Out of the things you don't necessarily *prefer* at the time, you can still create something that's not only *palatable* but downright *pleasurable* by what you add to it. It's the mix that matters!

The stories in this chapter speak to how it's possible to turn something unpleasant into something that can be *learned from* (or at least *laughed at*!) by virtue of *your attitude*. And, they're examples of how you can enjoy exceptional benefits in your life by simply choosing to look at things—particularly difficult things—from a slightly different perspective than your original vantage point. Just like someone did when they tasted rhubarb and helped transform it from something nearly inedible into something infinitely enjoyable. Your mind-set—and your life— deserve the same benefit of the doubt. And the results are well worth the effort. So, first, we'll talk pie, and then we'll talk perspective.

Strawberry-Rhubarb Pie

3 cups chopped rhubarb

3 cups sliced strawberries

1⅓ cups granulated sugar

¼ cup cornstarch

1 tablespoon lemon juice

¼ teaspoon cinnamon

Pastry for a double-crust 9-inch pie

1 egg, beaten (for glaze)

Sugar (for sprinkling over baked pie)

Line oven with foil or "drip catcher," or have a baking sheet handy to catch drips from the baking pie. Preheat oven to 425 degrees.

In a bowl, combine rhubarb, strawberries, sugar, cornstarch, lemon juice, and cinnamon. Spoon into a pastry-lined (unbaked) 9-inch pie plate. Top pie with pastry in preferred manner: either a lattice top or full pie pastry; slice to vent if you are using full top crust. Brush with beaten egg.

Bake for 15 minutes. Reduce heat to 375 degrees and bake for another 50–60 minutes (until crust is golden and rhubarb is tender when tested with a knife or toothpick).

Remove from oven, sprinkle with sugar, and enjoy while you ponder how you can change your perspective in life by adding different ingredients to things that, at the outset, seem unpalatable, but in the long run might produce something infinitely rewarding!

It's Not Always About You . . . But Sometimes, It Is!

One fine day, my three-year-old daughter, Malina, was engaged in a rather spirited debate with my husband about the merits of an afternoon pilgrimage to Chuck E. Cheese. As would any adult possessing an inkling of sanity (or a modicum of survival instinct), my husband felt sheer panic at the prospect of willingly imprisoning himself, toddler in tow, in an environment of both sensory and junk food overload. I admired his ability to maintain a calm façade, though I knew his mind was awash with images of exhausted, overwrought temper tantrums replete with sobbing and whining and the pulling of hair. And that was just the parents.

He began to display creative problem-solving skills that I've only seen on a few occasions in our years together (typically associated either with securing hard-to-book tee times or top-shelf martinis, or on his best days, a combination of the two). He offered a stunning array of alternatives that I felt, quite frankly, made a pretty good case for avoiding a run-in with "the big rat," as we have affectionately nicknamed Chuck. Games were mentioned, as was the park; a book-reading extravaganza; a trip to the mall or the kids' museum; a walk; a movie; and even miniature golf. Though she wasn't buying it at all, it made for a rather entertaining exchange, if you ask me.

After sparring for quite some time, Michael had finally had enough. He firmly said, "Malina, Daddy just doesn't *care* for Chuck E. Cheese." Wanting to school her in the finer points of negotiating win-win outcomes, he added, "I'd like us to decide together on something else we can do that we will *both* enjoy." Malina stopped for a moment to think, her mini mental wheels spinning like the eyes of children (and their parents) who have just exited the Chuck E. Cheese house of terror. She looked Michael squarely in the eyes, and said, "Daddy . . . it's not always about *you*. Sometimes, it's about *me*."

After nearly relieving himself on the family room floor in a fit of uncontrollable laughter, Michael granted, "She's got a point there." In a nod to her logical dexterity and unapologetic assertiveness, he conceded the win to his cherubic but worthy opponent. They marched off, tiny hand in massive one, to greet the rat. Indeed, it's not always about you. But sometimes it is. And it behooves you to know the difference.

A SLICE OF INSIGHT:
KNOWING WHEN IT REALLY *IS* ABOUT YOU

After witnessing the whole exchange firsthand, I got to thinking about the more noteworthy concept behind Malina's unintentionally funny comment—how we often blur the lines between knowing when something *is* and *is not* about *us*. This can cause serious blows to our self-esteem, stall our success, and significantly decrease our satisfaction in life. It serves us well to be clear about when it's *not* about us (as well as when it *is*).

> **W**hen you stop basing your self-concept and happiness on what other people think, you'll start truly living and feeling a heck of a lot better about most things in your life.

To start with, here are a few things that are *never*, under any circumstance, about *you*:

• **Other people's opinions.** All people are entitled to their own life experiences and their own perceptions. So, when someone disagrees with you or even judges you for something you have or haven't done, just remember, "It's not about you, it's about *them*." I think the title of Terry Cole-Whitaker's book *What You Think of Me Is None of My Business* sums up this concept beautifully. When you stop basing your self-concept and happiness on what other people think, you'll start truly living and feeling a heck of a lot better about most things in your life.

- **Other people's decisions and priorities.** While it would be so much easier if everyone *else's* decisions and priorities revolved around what was important to *us* (yes, I've advocated for this since I entered this world), the fact is that they all have their own needs, values, and schedules. Inevitably, for whatever reason, someone will decline your barbeque invitation (even though you prioritized her holiday party over your date night). Or, he'll opt out of supporting your kid's fund-raiser (even though you've had to set up a check register category to track your donations to his "charitable causes of the month"). Or, a colleague will neglect to return your call in a timely manner (even though she's acquired the coveted #4 slot on your speed dial list). In those cases, your *only* job is to remind yourself that their decision simply lines up with what's good for *them* right at that moment and wish them well. If we allow others to live their lives in ways that feel good to *them*, and when *we* do the same, everyone wins.

- **Unfortunate challenges and setbacks.** To politely paraphrase the old saying, "Stuff happens." Yet often, when things don't work out exactly as we had hoped, we tend to take things either personally, very personally, or überpersonally. We look for how and where we failed and then move on to how we let ourselves or others down. Sometimes we dub ourselves the official event planner for a wildly ornate pity party in our honor. The truth is, though, that usually there are a variety of reasons why things don't work out as planned. *Yes*, we need to accept responsibility for our actions and plan for how we'll navigate such things in the future, but we *don't* need to turn the whole experience into a psyche-bashing melodrama about how we "messed it all up . . . again." In these situations, *first* repeat the following mantra: *"This simply is what it is unless I choose to make it into something worse,"* and *then* decide to take *action* on what you *can* and to *release* your fixation on what you *can't* control. Your success (and your self-worth) will both benefit!

> First repeat the following mantra: "This simply is what it is unless I choose to make it into something worse," and *then* decide to take *action* on what you *can* and to *release* your fixation on what you *can't* control.

And now, for a few things that always *are* about you. These concepts are both deceptively simple and extraordinarily powerful. In any situation, it really *is* about you when you are doing the following four things:

- **Passionately and unapologetically living your values.** When you make your decisions and carry them out based on what *truly* matters to *you*, everyone (and everything) wins. That's because when you do this you are first in integrity with *yourself*, and then in integrity with *others* and *the world*. That's the foundation for making good decisions and feeling good about them in the process.

- **Joyfully seeking the greatest good you can contribute to your life and to the lives of others.** The key here is to be careful not to fall into the trap of trying to *please* others (which will always be a no-win situation). We are all here to serve in some way, and when we offer our greatest gifts to make the world a better place, we not only *feel* better but we also *enrich* others and *enhance* our shared life experiences.

- **Knowing with certainty that your happiness never depends on anyone else's opinions or approval.** This can be a tough one, especially because everyone wants to belong, to feel loved, and to be liked. When we meet with someone else's disapproval or judgment, it can feel like one (or all) of those things are in jeopardy. But ultimately, we all are entitled to our own opinions and outlooks, which are often colored by our unique history and perspective. Basing your happiness on someone else's perspective is about as effective as building your wardrobe around someone else's size and preferences—the result can be both uncomfortable *and* unflattering, to say the least.

> **B**asing your happiness on someone else's perspective is about as effective as building your wardrobe around someone else's size and preferences—the result can be both uncomfortable *and* unflattering, to say the least.

- **Following your heart about your best decision in any situation, and knowing with certainty that if others don't like it, that's their problem, not yours!** If you stay true to yourself and make the best decision with the information and resources you have at any given time, that's really the best you can do. Not everyone will like it or agree with it, and some people might even be pretty vocally opposed to it, but again, it's not *their* life (or decision); it's *yours*. Remember that we learn as much by what *doesn't* work as we do by what *does*, and that we learn on our own time line and in our own way . . . not vicariously through someone else's. Allowing other people to take accountability for *their* decisions and opinions while *you* take accountability for *yours* helps build stronger individuals and a stronger society.

> **W**hy not give yourself the grace and the space to ask yourself on a regular basis, "Is this *really* about *me*?" When it is, shout it from the mountaintop and celebrate your centeredness. When it's *not*, promptly release it and refocus on what's truly important to you.

So, how about it? Why not give yourself the grace and the space to ask yourself on a regular basis, "Is this *really* about *me*?" When it *is*, shout it from the mountaintop and celebrate your centeredness. When it's *not*, promptly release it and refocus on what's truly important to you . . . whether it's a trip to Chuck E. Cheese, a step toward a new job, a decision to marry, or a choice to forgo the company picnic. You know what you want . . . you know what you need . . . and with a little practice you can always clearly know when it *is* and when it's *not* about *you*!

MINDFULNESS BITE BY BITE:
ABOUT-FACE ON ABOUT YOU

1. When have you experienced a situation in which you mistook something for being "about you" when it really wasn't (and it ended up creating stress, disappointment, or other unpleasant outcomes)?

2. How might you re-script that experience to clearly describe which elements *were* and were *not* about you?

3. What can you do in similar situations in the future to help you do an "about-face" on what is "about you"? Why not commit to stepping back and objectively assessing what *is* and what is *not* about you?

The Winds of Change

On my first camping trip as an adult, I woke my first husband from a deep sleep during the middle of the night in a valiant effort to single-handedly roll our tent out of the way of an oncoming train. At the time, it didn't occur to me that it would be unlikely for a speeding locomotive to be bearing down upon us, threatening our very lives, in the middle of a national campground. But the howling wind and a rather vibrant dream state convinced me that our survival hung in the balance and that I needed to act swiftly to avert impending doom.

In a stunning display of physical prowess, I braced my feet against the nylon walls, stretched my arms out like a da Vinci sketch, and heaved the tent one full turn to the right. I unearthed all of the stakes in one mighty thrust and threw my husband like a rag doll out of his sleeping bag in a pile of human rubble, dazed, alarmed, and exceptionally annoyed. "What in the *hell* are you *doing*?" he sputtered. While my task seemed obvious to me at the time, I gasped, "I had to . . . get us . . . out of the way . . . of . . . that . . . train." And then I started to wake up.

After considerable reflection, I determined that it probably would have been much more effective to wake up *prior to* unleashing terror and carnage on our shelter for the night. But I guess everything's easier to see with a healthy dose of hindsight, a bit of consciousness, and the light of day (or the light of someone's burning gaze searing through you at 3 a.m.).

My husband's huge, wide eyes were startled, and he was seething. I think, in that moment, I may have witnessed the beginning of the end of our marriage. I whispered apologetically and sheepishly, trying to look cute and cuddly, "There's no train, is there?" Still, I covertly scanned the horizon for black smoke and strained to hear the chorus of a distant "chugga-chugga" through the stillness of the night. The only chugga-chugga I discerned was the adrenaline-fueled beating of my own heart and his labored breathing resulting from being awakened in such a shocking way. "NO, THERE ISN'T A *TRAIN*," he stammered through clenched teeth, as a down feather from his sleeping bag floated gently through the air, coming to rest on his lips. "AND NOW THERE ISN'T A *TENT* ANYMORE, *EITHER*!"

We spent an hour or so in the dark, braving the wind to piece together a makeshift refuge that would get us through the rest of the night. Although he would never admit it, *I* know that *he* knew that if there *had* been a train, I would have been a hero that night. I slept soundly with the knowledge that I could work wonders in the face of all odds (even when the odds were not only imagined but also inconvenient and inconsiderate). And he, I believe, slept with one eye open and one leg poised for escape for the remainder of the night . . . and perhaps for the remainder of our marriage.

A SLICE OF INSIGHT:
CHANNELING THE WINDS OF CHANGE

Okay. I know that this unfortunate but memorable little situation happened for a variety of reasons, including my tendency to sleepwalk in new and different situations, as well as environmental factors like the wind and darkness (not to mention the previously unrecognized tensions in my marriage). And I know that this particular set of conditions probably will never occur together again in my life (at least I can *hope* they won't). But I *do* know that I learned a few things about myself and about unforeseen circumstances that night (in addition to learning how readily I can overturn a well-secured tent in very short order in the event I ever need to in the future—I'm storing that one in my "just in case" file).

I learned that sometimes the winds of change can give you superhuman strength to tackle all sorts of things, welcome and unwelcome. It's best, though, to analyze whether the winds of change in your life are *actual* threats (like something that violates your values or undermines your happiness) or just *perceived* threats (such as things that are just *uncomfortable* because they're *different*, like new skills, schedules, or environments). In the case of the latter, it's best to give yourself a bit of time and space to get used to a new situation before taking radical action that might not serve your best interests (because trust me, that da Vinci pose can yield a wicked groin pull). A brief (and preferably conscious) analysis of your options can channel your most effective efforts into your most elegant outcomes.

So, rather than going on a reactionary rampage when faced with change, consider pausing and asking yourself, "Does this situation merit a significant investment of my precious time, energy, and resources?" The answer is probably no when you realize that you missed the homeowner's association meeting *again* this year (a simple calendar reminder for next year's will suffice). Or when your idea for the new project at work didn't receive a standing ovation (there are always more good ideas than opportunities to enact them). Or, when your dinner guests didn't touch your famous risotto (why question the good fortune of gourmet leftovers?).

> Rather than going on a reactionary rampage when faced with change, consider pausing and asking yourself, "Does this situation merit a significant investment of my precious time, energy, and resources?"

On the flip side, there are definitely times when your superhuman strength and fortitude might well be called for, such as when you've been downsized from your job and want (okay, *need*) to make a swift and purposeful transition into a new career. Or, when your retirement account has tanked and you want to make thoughtful decisions about reallocating your investments into a wealth-building vehicle rather than into fireplace kindling. Or when you and your partner have determined that your relationship isn't meeting your needs and you want to work together to restore it to its former grandeur. Your biggest priorities deserve the biggest share of your perspective.

Now, since we know that our minds can, without warning and with very little effort, readily distort the truth in a lot of different situations (as demonstrated in the aforementioned train fiasco), it's a good idea to watch out for thought patterns that might be erroneous at

> **U**ltimately, our best experiences happen when we harness the winds of change to achieve the results that we want in life, rather than allowing ourselves to be thrown about at their mercy.

best or counterproductive at worst. When you find that you are bracing yourself against the winds of change, remember that you often can choose to harness their power to create a wide array of positive outcomes. Sure, wind can *destroy* (as in the devastation that a hurricane can leave in its path). But it can also *build* (through the production of clean energy that fuels communities) and *move* (by filling sails that gently guide boats toward their destinations). Ultimately, our best experiences happen when we channel the winds of change to achieve the results that we want in life, rather than allowing ourselves to be thrown about at their mercy.

MINDFULNESS BITE BY BITE: WIND POWER

1. Where in your life has your mind made the winds of change into something they're not (perhaps in a relationship, job, financial situation, or personal development goal)?

2. What ideas do you have for how you can look at that situation in a fresh way that channels excitement or at least productive energy rather than sparking fear and frustration?

3. Is there a statement, image, or symbol you can identify to help remind you in the future to use the power generated by the winds of change to move your life *forward* rather than to *destroy* aspects of it?

Don't Freak Out

I headed to the foyer of a lovely hacienda in Puerto Vallarta, Mexico, to take a phone call. My siblings and I had saved for several years to spend our annual reunion enjoying a sunny seaside getaway together and it had been the week of a lifetime. I had mastered just three Spanish phrases that week: *"Dos cervezas, por favor"* ("Two beers, please"); *"No mas, gracias"* ("No more, thank you," when offered a fourth serving of the world's cheesiest chile rellenos); and *"Muy bueno"* ("Very good," when asked repeatedly how my vacation was going). These were really all the phrases I needed to get by in a setting where my only exercise consisted of walking from the pool to the dinner table, bar, or card game and back again. Twice a day I had to strain myself to ascend and descend the single flight of stairs to and from our room, but other than that, my muscles and my mind atrophied at a remarkably accelerated pace. I was in a certifiable Puerto Vallartan paradise.

My bliss was blindsided when I picked up the phone and the first words I heard through the static of those international phone lines were, "Don't freak out, Deenie. Everything's okay."

The voice was Amber's, one of my adult stepdaughters, calling from home, thousands of miles away, at a time that was expressly *not* our designated conversation hour. Chills shot through my body in the hundred-degree heat. Amber was watching our two-and-a-half-year-old, Malina, while we were on vacation. Since she has always been Malina's "second mom," she was the only reason I felt comfortable leaving my little pumpkin back in the States for a week while I enjoyed my first child-free getaway since becoming a parent. Amber and Malina were so close that I couldn't imagine anyone more worthy to entrust the well-being of my child to than a responsible, doting, and loving big sis. I didn't have a care in the world all week. Until that moment.

While my brain actually *did* register the words "Don't freak out," my mother's instinct went into autopilot, creating a rather graphic nuclear meltdown in my mind. Red lights flashed, alarms wailed, steam enveloped the frenzied scene in my gray matter, and I could have sworn I felt tiny people jogging down my neural pathways screaming, "RUN FOR COVER . . . SHE'S GONNA BLOW!" Halfway across the world, at least a day's travel away from my daughters, the words "Don't freak out" immediately registered on my perfectly calibrated freak-out instrument.

My heart raced, my head tingled, and my legs felt weak. All in a matter of seconds. I tried to remain calm, but all the little nuclear power plant workers in my brain donned biohazard suits and anxiously monitored erratic needles on my internal freak-o-meter. A blaring neon sign in my mind warned "Sector Four Contaminated! Commence psychic sanitation procedure immediately." Milliseconds seemed like millenniums as I pictured in graphic detail the wide array of crises that may have befallen one or both of my daughters while I lounged poolside in paradise. I tried to stay as calm and composed as I could, all the while imagining sinister plots being executed against my unsuspecting girls.

In the most responsive but nonchalant voice I could muster (which translated, I'm sure, to a tone of utter dread and sheer horror), I stammered, "Wh-wh-wh-what's going on, Amber?" Immediately sensing my impending loss of consciousness followed by the swift loss of my sanity, she quickly replied, "Mal and I are fine, but I thought you'd want to know that someone tried to break into the house while we were there last night. When I heard the noises, I got Mal, locked both of us in your room, and we called 911. The police came and checked everything out. They found where the people tried to get in, but they said everything's safe and secure now. We're both okay and the house is fine."

The little nuclear workers scattered to turn the release valves and the freak-o-meter started showing more reasonable levels of activity. The alarms subsided and a soft, reassuring voice oozed from the loudspeaker in my brain, announcing "All clear. All clear. The area has been secured. You may return to normal thinking." I exhaled so deeply that I think my rib cage may have imploded. Then I proceeded to learn more about what had happened and how Amber and Mal were doing. Thankfully, they were perfectly safe and sound after a most unsettling event. Amber just wanted to respectfully keep us informed so we wouldn't be surprised on our return. And, she wanted to do that in a thoughtful manner with a full assurance that everything was just fine. Thus, she led with, "Don't freak out." A well-intentioned move with a wildly unexpected impact.

A SLICE OF INSIGHT:
FORGO YOUR INNER FREAK

After the adrenaline wore off a few months (I mean *hours*) later, I reflected on why I had felt such an immediate, visceral response to those three words, when Amber was clearly and succinctly trying to assure me that everything was all right. I recalled an explanation I heard from a great speaker one time, who said, "The mind doesn't understand the word 'don't.' Since 'don't' can only be interpreted in reference to something *else*, your mind immediately fixates on whatever it's referring to in order to make sense of the statement. So, when you say 'Don't think about this,' or 'Don't focus on that,' your mind conveniently filters out the word 'don't' and expertly directs your attention to think about *exactly* what you're trying to *avoid*."

> When you say "Don't think about this," or "Don't focus on that," your mind conveniently filters out the word "don't" and expertly directs your attention to think about exactly what you're trying to avoid.

It's like the example, "Don't think of an orange whale with pink spots." The "don't" only has a function after you've clearly pictured the orange whale with pink spots in all its psychedelic glory, and then it directs you to somehow magically *erase* that image from your mind, usually by superimposing a big red circle with a slash through it over the top (thus making it even *more* colorful and memorable and even harder to ignore). And as you've guessed, my friends, the process of "un-thinking" a thought is nearly *impossible*. So there it sits, beckoning your attention until you divert your focus elsewhere. For me, those international phone lines served as a remarkably efficient translator, which morphed the words "don't freak out" efficiently into the phrase "FREAK OUT BIG-TIME RIGHT NOW WITH GREAT DRAMA AND FANFARE." All in a fraction of a second, and all without the benefit of a single conscious thought.

Why does this little story matter, aside from eliciting empathy and compassion from anyone else who's gone through a similar incident? As you may have guessed, there's a *practical* side to the tale as well. Quite simply, and quite contrary to conventional practice, it is far more productive to focus on what you *do* want in life, rather than what you *don't* want. While this sounds reasonable, and even easy to do, it actually can be quite a challenge because modern life is punctuated with don'ts of all sizes, shapes, and colors. Don't overeat . . . don't get too stressed . . . don't forget to floss . . . don't litter . . . don't be rude . . . don't shove that thing up your nose (more on this later) . . . don't go here, do that, be this, or have those. It's a veritable potpourri of "don't" every time we turn on the television or open up a newspaper. And it's an agenda of "don'ts" every time we sit down in a classroom or boardroom or examination room. *Don't worry*, though, there's a simple solution. Oops. You're right. Rather than "don't worry," why don't we focus on a practical alternative instead?

What kind of results do you suppose we could produce if we focused on the "dos" in life instead of the "don'ts"? Markedly better ones, I imagine. Since the mind filters out the "do" just as it does the "don't," you're left with the following messages: *eat* nutritious foods . . . breathe deeply and *relax* . . . *floss* every day . . . throw your trash in the can (better yet, recycle!) . . . *be kind* . . . leave that item in your hand (with its implied conclusion, "rather than wedging it up your nose"). It's an appeal to both our *logical* side and our love of *practical action* (after all, it's much easier to imagine taking *action* on something than it is to imagine what it means to *refrain from taking action* on something). It just makes more sense.

So, if you want to avoid obsessing about your unfinished to-do list at 3 a.m. rather than telling yourself, "*Don't* think about that overwhelming inventory of un-dones" (because, as we've all experienced, that's precisely what you will continue to ruminate on all night), redirect your thinking to what you *do* want, such as relaxation or peaceful sleep or efficient resolution to the items on your list (and, if needed, get up and write the list to assure your brain that you've taken *action*). Instead of instructing yourself *not* to fixate on the disappointment you experienced at work today, choose instead to methodically review your successes or list the things you're grateful for (and if it helps, record on paper so you can hold the proof in your hand and in your mind). Rather than telling yourself, "*Don't* consume the entire bag of Oreos," decide what you *will* do—truly savor an appropriate serving size (and remember the milk!). It's what we *do* (both in thought and in action) that creates momentum and results in our lives. And, since our decision on what to *do* comes from learning more about both the *situation* and our *options in it*, it's a good rule of thumb to translate your

> **I**t's much easier to imagine taking *action* on something than it is to imagine what it means to *refrain from taking action* on something. It just makes more sense.

> **I**t's what we *do* (both in thought and in action) that creates momentum and results in our lives.

"*Don't* freak out" into a far more productive "*Do* learn about" and then respond in a way that encourages freak-free living.

MINDFULNESS BITE BY BITE: FREAK-FREE LIVING

1. In what situation recently did you "freak out," even though you tried not to? What objectively happened prior to your emotional response?

2. How might you have prevented your freak-out by thinking *mindfully* rather than *reactively*?

3. What mental or physical steps might you take in the future to remain calm and thoughtful in an unexpected situation, thereby committing to freak-free living?

CHAPTER 3

Connection

To Serve and to Share

Don't Be a Connection Chicken; Accept the Pot Pie

I always assumed that I'd receive grand, life-changing revelations in the form of mystical dreams packed with complex symbolism and ethereal sound tracks. Or that I'd reach my personal aha moment about the workings of the universe at the hands of some ancient philosopher whose words reached me in *just* the right way at *just* the right time in my life. In fact, I'd probably even be inclined to welcome the kitschy amusement of a Magic 8 Ball delivering an entertaining combination of intrigue and inspiration. But I have to admit that I've been taken aback more times than I care to admit by the consistently mundane manner in which my most powerful insights have been presented to me. They're *usually* delivered by someone under the age of eight in the form of a traumatic brush with humiliation. But sometimes (on the most magical days) they're delivered dressed as timeless comfort foods wrapped in puff pastry. Go figure.

Such was the case, as you'll hear in the next story, with a certain chicken pot pie that helped the power of connection in my life. The delivery of said entrée stewarded into my life a whole new appreciation for the importance of both supporting and accepting support from others. Even though research clearly shows that social connection is one of the greatest determinants of health, happiness, and longevity, it seems that as a society we move further and further away from allowing that social fabric to wrap us in the warmth and comfort that it's intended to. We favor electronic tweets instead of in-person chats, and use voice-mail to communicate rather than our voices to truly connect. But fortunately it's still hard to Facebook a fresh-from-the-oven chicken pot pie, since a picture may be worth a thousand words but it's not worth a damn when you're hungry.

This chapter explores the importance of connection and the nuances involved in cultivating it in your life. Comfort food—whether it's chicken pot pie or anything else—is best served warm and shared with others. The same holds true for connection. Since I always favor eating first and educating second, we'll get started with a recipe for one of the best comfort foods of all time (good guess, chicken pot pie) and we'll end by exploring connection's role in centeredness, and thus, mindfulness.

Chicken Pot Pie

*2 cups peeled and diced potatoes (red, white, gold, or sweet
    potatoes, according to your preference)*
1 cup diced cooked carrots
6 tablespoons (¾ stick) unsalted butter
1 cup chopped yellow onion
½ cup chopped celery
Salt and pepper, to taste
6 tablespoons all-purpose flour
2 cups chicken stock
½ teaspoon poultry seasoning
½ teaspoon garlic powder
1 cup half-and-half (reduced fat is fine)
1 cup frozen peas
*2 cups shredded cooked chicken (baked, broiled, or poached
    chicken breast or rotisserie chicken, according to your
    preference)*
2 tablespoons parsley, optional
Pastry for a double-crust pie

Line oven with foil or "drip catcher," or have a baking sheet handy to catch drips from the baking pie. Preheat oven to 400 degrees. Grease a 9 x 9 or 9 x 13-inch baking pan and set aside.

Place potatoes in a large pot with enough salted water just to cover. Parboil for 6 to 8 minutes, until just tender. Drain and set aside.

Place carrots in a separate pot with enough salted water to cover. Parboil 4 to 5 minutes, until just tender. Drain and set aside.

Melt butter in a medium skillet over medium-high heat. Sauté onions and celery; add salt and pepper to taste, and continue to stir for 2 minutes. Add the flour to onion mixture and continue cooking 3 to 4 minutes, stirring occasionally. Add chicken stock, poultry seasoning, and garlic powder and bring the liquid to a boil.

Reduce heat to medium-low and simmer until the sauce begins to thicken, about 4 to 6 minutes. Stir in the half-and-half and continue to cook for another 4 minutes. Stir in potatoes, carrots, peas, chicken, and parsley. Add additional salt and pepper, as desired.

Line prepared baking pan with one of the piecrusts. Pour the filling into the pan and cover with the second crust. Seal the pie by tucking and crimping the edges and cut vents in the top crust.

Bake at 400 degrees until the crust is golden brown, approximately 25 to 30 minutes. Allow to cool 5 minutes prior to slicing.

Serve and share with others as you consider how something as simple as comfort food can be one instrument that helps us connect with others in meaningful ways.

Yes, Virginia, There *Is* a Lasagna Fairy

Just before my daughter Malina was born, I was given some of the most powerful and welcome advice I've ever received from my wonderful friend Kari. She pulled me aside one day after I had been polling people about the benefits of various breast pump models (aka "the mobile lactation station"), the late, great co-sleeping debate (aka "the marital intimacy prevention plan"), and the most essential baby gear (aka "I dream of Diaper Genie"). With a serious, almost stern tone to her voice, she said, "When you have this baby, people will offer you food. At the time, you won't want to impose. You won't want to be a burden. You'll try to politely say, 'Oh, we'll be fine,' and 'Please don't bother.' If you do nothing else, heed this advice: When people offer you food, you *take* it."

I'll admit that I was a bit taken aback by her emphatic urging, but since I love and respect her (and because she already had two kids at the time, so I figured she had the upper hand), I agreed. I'll admit I felt a bit sheepish saying yes to well-meaning women bearing casseroles, when I was an able-bodied person with a gourmet kitchen stocked with every imaginable piece of cooking paraphernalia. But, on Kari's sage advice, I responded to each offer with some version of, "We would really appreciate that," and "Thanks so much for thinking of us during this special time."

And then I had that baby. And I learned that she was right. Malina was my first baby and my first foray into an alternate universe that consisted of nothing but nursing, soothing, and in the very few, very short spells between those two activities, catching roughly one "z" (there were no strings of "zzzzzz's" to be had) before the whole cycle started again. There simply was no time to eat, much less to cook, despite that fact that this child was literally sucking the lifeblood out of me twenty-three out of every twenty-four hours and I needed sustenance. I will be eternally grateful to Kari for insisting that I graciously accept foodstuffs of any nature (though it did seem a bit much to use intimidation tactics to ensure I wouldn't turn down an offer of Chicken Divan or Auntie Pam's Cheesy-Ham and Potato Bake).

I said a brief prayer of thanks for good friends like Kari as I helped myself to yet another plate of one of those blessed casseroles about six days into life as a new parent. I noticed after consuming that fourth, and perhaps most fabulous, serving of pot pie that, through the magic of nursing, my tiny Malina smelled exactly like a savory little nine-pound chicken pot pie for the better part of her first week of life. To this day, every time I get a whiff of well-seasoned meats and vegetables enveloped in a light and flaky crust, I swear my bust increases by a full size. Who needs a miracle bra when a miracle casserole can do the same thing in a far more satisfying way?

And so we dined—and dined well, I might add. All due to Kari's sage advice. That's when I got to thinking about how women feel innately compelled to provide food for others during transitions and traumas, crises and celebrations. Word of a flu-ridden household, a relative's passing, the diagnosis of an illness, or the birth of a child turns us into Pyrex-wielding zombies droning, "Must . . . make . . . *shepherd's* . . . *pie*. Must . . . *bake . . . brownies*." We deliver comfort foods and good wishes in neatly packaged freezer bags and disposable roaster pans. New homes and new jobs provide an excuse to show up with a bottle of wine and chocolates in one hand and assorted cheese and garlic-laced goodies in the other. (Which, incidentally, is a revised food pyramid that I think we could all get behind using, if you ask me. Or get a bigger behind using. Maybe I'll need to rethink that.) While Hallmark wants us to say it with *greeting cards* and FTD wants us to say it with *flowers*, women intrinsically know that we're genetically programmed to "say it with food." Or better yet, we don't have to *say* it . . . we can *savor* it . . . with food.

In fact, we're so skilled and committed to the practice that I even had one friend who literally broke into my home after Malina was born to deliver her world-famous lasagna. She had been duly warned by my coworkers that "if and when the *baby* sleeps, the *parents* sleep," so she didn't want to take a chance that she'd wake either party by ringing the doorbell. When we didn't respond to her entirely inaudible knocks at the front door (we spent most of our time upstairs staring at the baby for hours nonstop when we weren't consuming massive quantities of chicken pot pie), she decided to skulk around to the back of our house, break in through a slider door, and leave a fresh (and fabulous) lasagna in the refrigerator.

I stumbled downstairs later that day, ready to rifle through the fridge for something to put an end to my unplanned starvation diet, and what to my wondrous eyes did appear, but a full tray of lasagna, nestled amongst the beer. I blinked a couple of times. "Honey," I yelled, "is there such a thing as a Lasagna Fairy?" "Whu . . ." Michael mumbled, shoveling a bite of chicken pot pie into his mouth. "Okay. When we went upstairs, there *wasn't* a lasagna in the fridge. And now there *is* a lasagna in the fridge. Does that mean there's a Lasagna Fairy?" "Hmmph," he replied, mouth half full of his next bite. He raised his eyebrows and shrugged his shoulders as if to say, "I dunno, but who cares where it comes from, as long as it's good!"

I thought it was pretty cool to be visited by a pasta-packing pixie, which my sleep-deprived mind determined looked exactly like Rachael Ray. Years later, I did confirm the existence of that out-of-sight-Italian-sprite. The Lasagna Fairy again visited when my son, Carsten, was about six months old. He'd contracted a massive double ear infection, the pain of which was only periodically masked by the unfortunate fits associated with truly epic stomach flu. It was the kind of illness only a mother would stick around for (and, truth be told, even I felt like a prisoner of . . . gore . . . and repeatedly considered tunneling out, but it would have taken too much energy to do that given my steady diet of nothing but saltines and breakfast cereal for days).

Fortunately for him (and, of course, unfortunately for me) my husband was out of town during the whole incident. By the time I took Carsten to the ER, where they poked and prodded him in the most undignified way, culminating with the insertion of an IV into his chubby little arm, Michael was booked on a flight home. But since I'd borne the brunt of the sleepless nights and the festival of body fluids, I was starting to lose most of my faculties (which I guess assumes I had some to start with, and I'm not so sure that's correct). I officially started to hallucinate.

The next day, my wavering resolve to power through this until Michael got home gave way to a flood of tears when my friend Debbie called. I shared a summary of the past few days, which sounded something like: ". . . up all night every night . . . so tired . . . won't stop crying . . . can't make it go away . . . have to hold him 24/7 . . . he's so chubby my wrists are giving out . . . do they do wrist transfusions? . . . or transplants? . . . or houseplants? . . . because I can't even pick him up anymore . . . the Republicans must be behind this . . . I see dead people." The phone went eerily silent and she reassuringly said, "Hold on, honey. I'll be there soon."

Within hours, she met me with a bag filled with goodies. Fresh flowers poked out of the top and I found myself on a gourmet treasure hunt. My mood perked up immensely when I found a colorful salad with balsamic dressing, freshly baked artisan bread, and an assortment of rich, dark chocolates. Next came the requisite lasagna, ready to be warmed. My recovery was imminent. And I somehow felt a decrease in my resentment toward Michael for being out of town, the Republicans for whatever part they played, and the dead people who had infiltrated my hallucinations the night before. I suddenly felt revived and almost broke into a *Sound of Music* remix of "My Favorite Things." My wrists mysteriously regained their strength, allowing me to clap excitedly while jumping up and down like a kid at Christmas when I laid my eyes on the last item in the bag: a fabulous bottle of wine. I don't know about you, but to me, nothing says "Stop dangling on the precipice of a nervous breakdown" like a good bottle of Chianti.

I phoned Michael. "Honey," I gushed, "there most definitely *is* a Lasagna Fairy and *now* she brings wine and chocolate with a Martha Stewart–inspired tablescape and a range of bistro-style accompaniments. If we keep having babies there's no *telling* what she's capable of!" I'm not exactly sure what he thought, but he spoke to me in a very soft, reassuring tone and managed to catch an even earlier flight home. We shared the lasagna but the Chianti and chocolate were all mine. I'd earned them.

A SLICE OF INSIGHT:
OF FAIRIES AND FRIENDSHIPS

The Lasagna Fairy stands for everything noble women do in service to others. We go out of our way to ease suffering and to nurture those in need. We band together to foster health, healing, and happiness without expecting anything in return. And we do it with, among many other wonderful things, *food*. Now, I know what you might be thinking: "Hold on, Deanna. Sometimes a lasagna is just a lasagna, right?" Not in this case. In this realm, lasagna symbolizes connection and compassion and comfort. It's a physical manifestation of friendship. It's four or five layers of warm, bubbly love. Long live the woman who's gotta share her ricotta!

Seriously, though, you can't argue with the research that says that "female bonding" helps make women more resilient and more satisfied, healthier and happier. Our brains and bodies crave linking up with other women just like they crave that lasagna. And when you merge the pals and pasta, doesn't everyone win?

There's actually a term for the healing power of female connections. It's called the Tend and Befriend theory, and it was coined by Shelley Taylor, professor of psychology at UCLA. Taylor's pioneering research has demonstrated the powerful way in which social relationships serve as protective factors against stress. Her Tend and Befriend theory suggests that, when faced with crises or challenges, women are hard-wired to *tend* to others (their young, their families, those in need) and to *befriend* other women to help them navigate challenging situations and life stressors. In short, we *engage* with others both to *endure* hardship and to *enrich* our lives.

> In short, we *engage* with others both to *endure* hardship and to *enrich* our lives.

These "coping connections" have both physical and psychological benefits. *Physical* benefits include the release of oxytocin, a hormone that causes a profound sense of relaxation and that conveniently helps neutralize stress hormones in the body (think of it as kind of an antacid for upset emotions rather than upset stomachs). *Psychological* benefits include far more than just a sense of camaraderie or an impressive social calendar, though who'd turn that down? No, when we connect in meaningful ways, we reap the lasting impact of comfort and support, creative problem-solving, and even the collective stewardship of ideas and resources during tough times. And all this from the seemingly insignificant gestures of a phone call or a girls' night out, a knitting group or a homemade meal.

> When we connect in meaningful ways, we reap the lasting impact of comfort and support, creative problem-solving, and even the collective stewardship of ideas and resources during tough times.

There's an important consideration to think about in regard to the Tend and Befriend theory. As women, it seems that we are often inclined to do a heck of a lot more *tending* than *befriending*. Most women I know have struggled with the fact that they often serve others at the expense of both their own self-care and their time with other women. What are the first two things that get sacrificed when your schedule blows up or your to-do list multiplies exponentially? Time for self and time for friends. The phenomenon has reached nearly epidemic proportions for the women who attend my events and read my books. How about you? It's time to start adding yourself to the top of the list of

> It's time to start adding yourself to the top of the list of people you care *about* and care *for*. When you do that, you magnify your ability to both *give* and *live*.

people you care *about* and care *for*. When you do that, you magnify your ability to both *give* and *live*.

It seems like there might be value in not only inviting the Lasagna Fairy to visit friends in crisis but also calling on friends (including yourself) who simply crave the ongoing connection of a book group or breakfast bunch, a coffee klatch, or an exercise class. Yes, like all of us, that nimble little sprite is capable of wearing a few different hats. She's a champion of both *prevention* (staving off stress and enhancing well-being *now*) as well as *intervention* (swooping in to serve when things aren't going well *later*). So why not beckon her a little more often or consider donning your own wings to deliver a little stress relief to someone you care about (yourself included)?

MINDFULNESS BITE BY BITE: COMFORT FOOD FOR THE SOUL

1. Take a look at your schedule and/or your to-do list. Does time for self-care or time for friends appear on your calendar and/or list at regular, healthy intervals?

2. How can you make time and space in your life to engage with your friends more *often*, particularly when one of you is *not* in desperate need? (Perhaps consider regularly scheduled dates for coffee, girls' night out, or pedicures.)

3. How can you serve up your own "comfort food for the soul" by looking for ways to nurture *yourself* on a regular basis? Why not commit to adding yourself to your to-do list so you're sure *you* will be a priority just like everything else?

A Presidential Mishap

When my husband, Michael, and I got together, we merged households and moved into my home on the opposite side of town from his. This made it necessary for my stepdaughter Rhiannon to change school districts during her junior year in high school. Because of differences in the curriculum, Rhee ended up sharing a couple of classes with seniors, including a political science course. One assignment tasked her with writing a research essay on former president Nixon, which she was required to present as a formal speech, complete with audiovisual aids, in front of her classmates.

She spent the weekend writing her paper and crafting her poster board display. We read the paper and were duly impressed. It was well written, detail oriented, and definitely "A"-quality work. The display was creative and comprehensive, and it included the requisite pictures of President Nixon waving from the plane and shaking hands with Elvis. She had done a stellar job and we told her so. We sent her off to school certain that she would ace her presentation.

That evening, Michael and I picked her up from her after-school job with my visiting friend, Deb, in tow. When we pulled up to the store, Rhee was sitting on the curb out front with a rather strange look on her face. She silently slid into the car, fastened her seatbelt, and settled in. She hadn't said a word, so we hit her with the question we'd been dying to ask, "So, how did it *go*?" She glanced up, her wide eyes incredulous and full of dread, and blurted out, "Did you know that President Nixon is *dead*?"

A thousand thoughts flooded my mind in the seconds that followed. I knew that she had given her presentation not only in front of a group of teenagers but also in front of a group of *seniors*. I knew from experience that public speaking can be challenging even in front of the best of audiences. I knew that puberty ushers in many things, among which are fragile adolescent egos and a peer group that can be either compassion-challenged or ridicule-rich and, at times, both. So, I surmised this would be a critical time for me to say and do *just* the right thing to help our sweet girl recover from whatever debacle had taken place in that classroom.

Before I could respond, though, with what would have been the gold standard of all parental pep talks, my friend Deb, a full-fledged adult complete with a shiny college degree, who should have *known* that President Nixon had died *several* years earlier, squealed, "*No!* What *happened*? Was it a *stroke*?" She said it in one of those really high-pitched voices barely audible to human ears, but that effectively beckons all of the dogs in the neighborhood to come running. It was nearly impossible to discern what she was saying but we sensed that perhaps she was ever so slightly surprised about *something*.

So I responded in the only way I could in that delicate situation. I laughed. I laughed hard and loud and long, crescendoing to what I believe was a most unbecoming snort. I swear I lost a number of bodily functions in that moment, which I won't go into here, but suffice it to say that the laughter was not just *uncontrollable* but also entirely *contagious*. All four of us spent the next five minutes doubled over, alternately holding our midsections and wiping tears from our eyes. When we finally contained the outburst we stammered, "What on earth . . . *happened*?"

"Well," she said, "I gave my presentation, which went really well. I'm thinking to myself, 'Hey, not bad . . . you nailed it.' Then, during the question-and-answer time, this guy from the back of the room raises his hand and says, 'S'cuse me, Rhee, but isn't President Nixon *dead*?'" Now, Rhee is a fairly self-assured young woman, well-poised in situations like these, so she responded directly and with certainty, "Oh, no, no, no. He's alive. I think he's living in New York. I think he's writing books now." Evidently she'd come up just a bit shy in her chronological detailing of President Nixon's life and times, and you can bet that her classmates were prepared to show her the error of her ways, judging by the shuffling and whispering going on in the room.

Her teacher recognized that the situation would be careening downhill very rapidly very soon, so he stepped in to offer his comments. "No, Rhiannon. President Nixon has indeed passed away." Turning to her poster board display, he pointed to the picture of Elvis and President Nixon shaking hands, and said, "Now, *Elvis* may still be alive. In fact, I think that someone may have seen him at a convenience store last week, but we *do* have evidence that President Nixon is no longer with us. But, *great* presentation. You can take your seat now." She somehow managed to survive the humiliation and was able to make it through the rest of the school year without another error of omission that grave and, surprisingly, without too much damage to either her psyche or her social calendar.

But she hasn't been quite so lucky on the home front. In

fact, every time a major political story breaks, I dial her up and ask, in my most self-assured voice (which I mastered by listening to hers, of course), "Hey, Rhee. Uh, what do you think former president Nixon would think of that? Do you think he would have a comment or insight on it? Could you phone him and ask, since I know you seem to know his whereabouts pretty well?" She responds with colorful language and asks me if the following noise sounds like a phone hanging up. And interestingly, it always does.

A SLICE OF INSIGHT:
A MEANINGFUL MISFORTUNE

What a gift laughter can be. It entertains and energizes us, often when we need it most. It has the power both to distract and to connect, with the benefit of providing both healing and hope. And it's often most powerful when it's least expected. I truly believe that, when dispensed with joy and respect, laughter is one of the most potent cures for what ails individuals, families, organizations, and communities.

> What a gift laughter can be. It entertains and energizes us, often when we need it most. It has the power both to distract and to connect, with the benefit of providing both healing and hope. And it's often most powerful when it's least expected.

Sure, laughter has physical benefits. It releases endorphins, the body's natural opiates, which create feelings of well-being and relief from pain. It exercises the heart, lungs, and those all-important abdominal muscles. It's a sleep aid, immune booster, and a natural way to reduce food cravings (no prescription or willpower required). And it decreases blood pressure and promotes healing, among many other things. A little mirth also goes a long way toward psychological health. It counteracts stress hormones in the body, eases symptoms of depression, and helps reduce anxiety. It also distracts us from negative emotions like anger, guilt, and (thankfully) embarrassment. Laughter has long been known as "the best medicine" for good reason.

But who knew that the benefits of laughter could extend so far beyond its role as the great entertainer and the great healer? It continues to become more and more apparent that laughter is also the great *connector*. The field of social intelligence suggests that we actually make and remake memories consistently throughout life, rewiring our brains through the impact of our personal experiences *and* through our shared interactions with one another. So, when we connect with one another in laughter about a memorable event (even one of presidential proportions), not only does it release neurotransmitters—those feel-good chemicals in our bodies and brains that make us more likely to remember the incident—but it actually helps solidify a *collective* memory of the experience, where each player contributes a certain amount of their recall to paint the full picture of what actually happened. When we laugh together, we literally co-create both our experience at that moment and our shared history.

> When we laugh together, we literally co-create both our experience at that moment and our shared history.

Imagine the potential we have to alter our *memory* of something in a positive way, and (even more significant) to influence our *future* actions based on that memory using something as simple . . . and enjoyable . . . and inexpensive . . . as a shared laugh. What a powerful notion that is! So, in this case, Rhee *could* have experienced any number of unpleasant outcomes after this embarrassment, not the least of which could have been a self-concept suited to wiping one's muddy shoes on after a big rainstorm or an incurable phobia of public speaking (and/or public figures of historical significance). Instead, through the magic of laughter, she was *distracted* (if only briefly) from her pain and, more important, *connected* to people who care about her, through a lighthearted collective memory of the incident. Now, I'm sure that on occasion she entertains whether it would be preferable to have only her *own* memory of the event rather than our *shared* one (mainly during presidential debates, during which we regularly consult her for insider feedback on how the candidates are doing). But, the fact remains that she is radically healthier—physically, psychologically, and socially—because we laughed with her that day. And the best thing is that we can regularly create those kinds of outcomes for ourselves and others by sharing laughter and connection, even in the most challenging times.

MINDFULNESS BITE BY BITE: CATASTROPHES THAT CONNECT

1. Are there times when you have endured something unfortunate or unpleasant that you had a hard time getting over (and an even harder time laughing about?)

2. Can you identify one or two elements from those times that offered you an opportunity to learn, to connect, or to build meaning in your life . . . or that afforded you the opportunity to laugh (even a little)?

3. How might you program your perspective to seek out either comedy or connection (or both!) in the catastrophes of the future?

An Identity Crisis

I adore my husband. I really do. He's just about everything a woman could want in a man and more. He's funny. Handsome. Smart. A great dad. A savvy business partner. A self-directed-garbage-taker-outer. The whole package. Definitely a keeper. And yet with all of his many, *many* strengths, there are certain days when I find him to be *less enlightened* than I feel he should be, particularly on the days when he is delayed either in recognizing when *he* is wrong and *I* am right or when he fails to remedy said situation promptly enough and with sufficient remorse.

On the day in question, Michael had not yet seen the light about whatever egregious error he had made, and I was tired of bodily dragging him to the light switch only to fume as he stumbled away in utter darkness. Now, because I am simply mad *about* my husband, I typically don't feel the need to share his faults with others on a regular basis unless I am overwhelmingly mad *at* him. On this day, I needed a safe outlet for my righteous indignation. I needed a willing venting partner, but not just anyone. I needed someone I could *trust*.

I wanted to confide in someone who would not only *sympathize with me* but also *fully commiserate with me with an unprecedented level of discretion*. This person needed to be someone who respected the sacredness of my marriage and my deep, abiding love for my husband, and who would maintain full confidentiality about his unfortunate but understandable flaws (after all, he's human). It needed to be someone who would *never* overstep her bounds by violating the "girlfriends' grievance against guys commandment," which reads, "Thou shalt not talk trash about my loved one, even if I do." You can *agree* with my complaints, and even sprinkle appropriately inflected "Oh, no he *didn't*s" and "You've *got* to be *kiddings*!" but you may *not*, under any circumstance, share your own opinions of his regrettable shortcomings. That's just in poor taste. And besides (mark my words), I'll remember it.

So, from my list of trusted confidantes, I called one of my sisters, Michelle, knowing with certainty that she would validate my every complaint without once offering personal comments on Michael's charming character flaws. While all of my other sisters would have been equally effective as confidantes that day, Michelle lives in close geographic proximity, so I figured that my rage would remain more intact over the shorter distance between cell phone towers. When Michelle answered the phone, because we're both busy people, I launched right in so I wouldn't waste her time, nor mine, with small talk. I wanted to land my "flight of many complaints" on her runway and dump my baggage for her to cart around on my behalf for a while (like a skilled porter who would never dream of diverting your favorite unmentionables to Kuala Lumpur as payback for a skimpy tip).

I began with, "*If* I hack my husband into tiny pieces . . . *will* you help me scatter his remains throughout the Pacific Northwest?" There was a pause at the other end of the line, as I imagined there would be. I expected as much and wasn't offended in the slightest. After all, this was a pretty significant request and I knew she'd have to consider the potential repercussions of aiding and abetting me. I knew that she really liked Michael and that would make her decision even more difficult, but I also knew that blood was thicker than water. Or I guess I *hoped* it was. And if blood wasn't thicker than water, I would move on to determining whether pomegranate martinis were, because I was prepared to spring for a round or two after she proved her loyalty. Through that brief silence, I could sense she was on the urge of an emphatic, though anxious, "OF COURSE I WILL!" because that's what sisters do. Or at least that's what *my* sisters do. So I continued.

". . . Because I watch *CSI* and I know that the investigators will be looking for trace evidence. You're the smartest person I know and I need your help covering it up." As I prepared myself for the meaty part of the conversation—the planning, brainstorming, sinister meetings in dark alleys (or over dark coffee in local espresso shops, at least)—another quiet delay ensued on the other end of the line. For a moment, I felt badly about putting her in this position. Would she ask the same of me? Would she put my life and freedom in jeopardy, too, to express her own temporary bout of hostility? "No," I said to myself, "she wouldn't. But *I* would. And I *have*. And now *the ball's in her court*. I'll soon know the extent of her love for me."

After another uncharacteristically long pause, I eagerly awaited her affirmative, "Count me IN!" because, honestly, you've reached a pretty lofty position on the ladder of friendship when you're asked to help dispose of a body. There's a linear progression that includes collecting your friend's mail during her vacation, followed by feeding her pets when she's away, which leads to babysitting her children when needed. But disposing of a body is in a class all itself. It's really the pinnacle of accomplishment that indicates you have truly "arrived" as a friend. I knew she'd be touched. Honored, in fact. And so there I sat, patiently expecting her emphatic, "YES! I will help you!" to echo through the phone lines. Instead, what I heard was, *"Aunt Deanna, I don't think that's a good idea."*

I had one of those moments when my neurons didn't fire quite as they should. Or, more likely, they misfired, went up in flames, and then dissolved into a heap of charred ashes somewhere in the folds of my gray matter. Michelle's voice sounded different. Younger, and more innocent. Almost like a prepubescent male. How strange the extent to which unchecked annoyance can affect our senses! I continued to process for a few seconds to sort out the response I *anticipated* compared to the one I had *received*. And then it hit me: The voice I heard in response to my plea for help concealing the dismembered remains of my husband's lifeless body was that of my nephew Jacob, eight years old at the time.

I panicked, not something I often do. My heart started pounding. I donned my most syrupy lovey-dovey voice, the one reserved for cute babies, cuddly puppies, and fluffy kitties, and stuttered, "Uh . . . Jacob, honey . . . uh . . . is your mommy there? Can I talk to your mommy, please?" with that final please trailing off into an alarmingly high-pitched timbre. Michelle quickly piped up in that "mother of all voices that means business," "Jacob, I've got it." And I heard the other extension click. Yes, she had answered the other phone extension at the same moment as my nephew, and I just couldn't hear Jacob's harmonizing "hello" through the chorus in my mind singing about Michael's wrongdoings in three-part harmony.

I spent the next ten minutes anxiously asking Michelle to relay messages to Jacob, like one of those old telegraph relay systems. "Dear Jacob. Stop. Aunt Deanna was just kidding. Stop. Aunt Deanna would never do anything to harm Uncle Blocky. Stop. Aunt Deanna is *so* sorry if she offended you in any way. Stop. And Aunt Deanna thinks that you should *never* answer the phone again. And I mean *stop*." I heard my sister relay each and every message to Jacob with calm repose until the last one, which she simply relayed as, "Mommy loves you. Now go outside and play."

So, I'd worked my magic on yet *another* youngster's impressionable mind, all for the purpose of gaining reinforcements in my little battle with Michael. With ill-constructed rules of engagement the skirmish yielded collateral damage in the form of Jacob's significant anxiety levels in the coming months. I noticed that every time I spoke with him by phone he was uncharacteristically—and I mean *disturbingly*—pleasant. He'd engage in trivial chitchat while waiting for the right moment to gingerly ask, "So . . . Aunt Deanna . . . uh . . . how's Uncle Blocky doing? Is he doing okay? I . . . uh . . . Haven't seen him in a while. Is he *around*? Can I . . . uh . . . *talk* to him?" It was always this uncomfortable mix of nervousness and foreboding, with an undertone of "I know what you did last night." I'm not sure who was more taken aback by the whole interchange, Jacob or myself, but I do know that I learned (and rather quickly, I might add), just how important it is to *know with whom you are speaking prior to voicing anything incriminating*. A case of mistaken identity can create complications in a number of ways. Just ask me. Better yet, ask Jacob.

A SLICE OF INSIGHT:
IDENTITY CRISIS RESPONSE TEAM

It's no secret that we need other people to help us stay healthy, happy, and (as in the above story) on the favorable side of the law. Research proves that people who enjoy a rich network of social connections live longer, are more satisfied, manage stress better, and have greater well-being on many levels than people who don't. And isn't it true that when we're facing difficulties we typically turn to others (often other women) to support us and to strategize with us, to console us and to get creative with us?

> **R**esearch proves that people who enjoy a rich network of social connections live longer, are more satisfied, manage stress better, and have greater well-being on many levels than people who don't.

So, on one hand, when I called Michelle (my sister and trusted confidante) to unload my frustration about Michael (my beloved though imperfect husband), I was simply following my genetic programming to do so. I knew that through our connection, she would be able to help "talk me down" more effectively (and probably more enjoyably) than I would be able to do myself. I knew she would help dissipate the emotional charge of the situation with a sympathetic ear and a sassy sense of humor. We all benefit from a little catharsis when the going gets tough, and one of the best ways to purge those emotions is to share them with a willing listener.

On the other hand, there are a couple of critical things to think about when you're seeking consolation and connection during stressful times. First, research does indeed show that when you productively purge those negative thoughts, it can significantly improve how you feel both in mind and in body. In fact, you can experience a swift decrease in feelings of anxiety and depression, as well as an immediate immune system benefit just by journaling about a particular hardship or sharing it with someone else. The critical factor to remember, though, is that *more is not better*. An *opposite* effect can happen when you share "too much of a bad thing." Since the mind and body don't know the difference between *experiencing* something and *vividly thinking* about it, if you recount complaints and grievances over and over, your brain and body believe that these slights are happening repeatedly, so they respond by *boosting* stress hormones rather than what you really want to do—*reduce* them.

> Since the mind and body don't know the difference between experiencing something and vividly thinking about it, if you recount complaints and grievances over and over, your brain and body believe that these slights are happening repeatedly, so they respond by boosting stress hormones rather than what you really want to do—reduce them.

The best rule of thumb when connecting with others to survive a challenging time is to follow two simple guidelines, referred to as the "PS" and the "BS." The *PS* means to "purge sufficiently" and then seek resolution, reframing, or release. Your goal here is to share the issue, process it thoroughly, and brainstorm ways to *solve the problem* if you can (resolution). In the event you can't solve it, your next step is to *change the way you look at it* (reframing) in order to reduce stress or redirect your thinking toward more productive topics. Sometimes it can be valuable to seek professional help with this process from a therapist, mentor, or spiritual advisor. And finally, when you feel prepared and ready to move on, you can simply make a decision to *let it go* (release). If you repeatedly reorient yourself to the negative emotion (rather than its resolution, reframing, or release), you'll likely feel far *more* stress than *relief*.

So those steps are the *PS*, but what's the *BS*? *BS*, in my opinion, is just as important (rest assured, fair readers, it's a markedly different BS than you're used to). I encourage you to learn a lesson from my "identity crisis" with Michelle and Jacob—always be sure that you verify the identity of the person from whom you are seeking support. Your ability to heal and to find hope again is in part dependent upon your ability to *connect with the right person in the right way at the right time*. That's why the concept of BS is so critical. You must *bond safely (BS)*, my friends, by always confirming that your pleas for help and guidance are heard by the intended recipient. This is important not only to avoid cases of mistaken identity—like mine—but also to be sure that you are turning to someone who will be able to listen, understand, and (when asked) provide wise counsel.

> **Y**our ability to heal and to find hope again is in part dependent upon your ability to connect with the right person in the right way at the right time.

There are many reasons why you *wouldn't* want to share certain things with certain people, including if they've experienced recent crises or a previous loss that would make it painful for them to attend to yours (for instance, a person who's recently been downsized from her ideal job may not be the best person to field complaints about your workload or boss). Or, if you're not convinced of the person's ability to exercise discretion and good judgment about what you've shared (his history of detailing the private lives of everyone in your neighborhood might be a good clue). Or, if you're not completely certain she has *your best interests in mind* (beware the false confidante who will share your personal details

> **U**ltimately, you simply want to feel secure that you are engaging with a trusted friend who will *help*, not *hinder*, the situation.

with others to get ahead in her career or to boost an unhealthy self-concept). Ultimately, you simply want to feel secure that you are engaging a trusted friend who will *help*, not *hinder*, the situation. Otherwise, you'll have a completely *different* set of stressors to deal with (as I did in my case of mistaken identity), and who needs that?

MINDFULNESS BITE BY BITE: TEAMWORK FOR TRAUMAS

1. Think of a challenge or a stressor that you've struggled with recently, one that you haven't been able to resolve or release on your own.

2. List a variety of people in your life whom you would feel comfortable turning to in times of need, whether you need empathy or support, a listening ear, or a good laugh. (Remember, you may identify different *people* who can fill different *needs* for you at different *times*.)

3. Consider sharing your stressor or struggle with one person on that list, taking care to observe the PS and BS guidelines—*purge sufficiently* (share it once, then move on to resolving, reframing, or releasing it), and *bond safely* (always verify you're sharing with the intended—and most appropriate—person!).

PTER 4

tability

he Product . . . Not Perfection

Heavy Sigh, Then Mud Pie

Sometimes things just don't work out exactly like we had planned. Whether it's a pie recipe or life, occasionally some of our outcomes aren't the stuff of dreams (let's be honest, at times they easily could be classified as nightmares), but they still enrich our lives in one way or another. The whole notion always makes me think of mud pie, because every time I'm in a situation where I've "got mud on my face," mortified by the newest manner in which I've humiliated myself (and *trust* me, those instances are far more frequent than I wish they were), I figure it's a probably a good time for a heavy sigh and some mud pie instead of wasting my time dwelling on it. In fact, I'm typically far more likely to dwell on anything that is sinfully rich than on my sins, per se.

This particular combination of things—a deep breath and a deep-dish slice of pure frozen fabulosity—gives me the respite I need to collect myself, learn what I need to learn from the incident, and move on. And mud pie gives me the energy to do it. (Okay, more from a *psychological* than a *physical* standpoint but whatever works, right?) Even more appropriate is that mud pie is one of those tasty treats that can be thrown together haphazardly; and even when it looks like a train wreck (kind of like life does at times), no one really cares because it's still so exquisitely satisfying (also like life most of the time). It's a great message to remember that sometimes the process, and even the product, of life (and, of course, pies) can be kind of messy, but ultimately they still produce something worth savoring. There's much to be said for the way that some of our most striking *imperfections* can provide us with the perfect opportunities to make *progress* in life.

The following tales focus on *adaptability*—being able to recover from setbacks with a sense of humor, and to learn important lessons in the most humble of ways (even when we feel like we're quite humble enough already, thank you). And if we can enjoy a *pie* that doesn't necessarily look like a work of art but still *tastes* like one, it seems that we can lead a *life* that doesn't always look like a work of art but still *feels* like one. Let's start with the pie and move on to the sigh.

Mud Pie

½ cup peanut butter

1 prepared chocolate cookie crumb or graham-cracker crust
    (purchased)

1 pint chocolate ice cream, softened

⅔ cup chopped Nutter Butter cookies

1 pint cookies and cream ice cream, softened

2 full Twix bars (4 sticks), chopped

1 pint coffee ice cream, softened

Chocolate sauce or hot fudge sauce

Caramel sauce, optional

Toasted almonds, optional

Whipped cream, optional

Spread the peanut butter in the bottom of the prepared crust. Cover with the softened chocolate ice cream and top with Nutter Butter cookies.

In a mixing bowl that is the same diameter (or slightly smaller) as the pie crust (typically roughly 8–9 inches, depending on crust size), place the softened cookies and cream ice cream in the bottom of the bowl and even out the top. Sprinkle with chopped Twix bars.

Place both the pie plate and the bowl in the freezer for 1 hour, then take the bowl out and top with softened coffee ice cream. Return to the freezer for 1 hour.

Remove both the pie plate and the bowl from the freezer. Spread the chocolate sauce topping over the frozen Nutter Butter cookies. Float the bowl of ice cream in warm water for 1–2 minutes to loosen the ice cream, then invert it over the pie plate (on top of the hot fudge) so that the ice cream becomes the top layer (it will be a big "mound" on top of the pie).

Garnish with more chocolate sauce or hot fudge, and add caramel sauce, toasted almonds, and whipped cream as desired.

Enjoy a heavy sigh and a slice of mud pie any time you

need to remind yourself that it's the *process* and the *product*, not *perfection*, that we're after in this life!

A Turn for the Worse

At age thirty, I decided to return to my roots as a classical dancer and enrolled in an adult ballet class at a studio near my office. A friend and I donned our leotards, stretched our emerging wisps of gray into buns, and headed to the barre. Even as a teenager, though I was a fairly accomplished dancer, I wasn't one of those lanky, willowy ballerinas who looked like a reed swaying in the wind. Instead, I was their slightly rotund, fluffy counterpart who resembled tumbleweed gracefully meandering about the prairie. And, after twelve years, my tumbleweed had expanded a bit in diameter. I spent a few months getting to know my body again, or at least getting to know the new additions to it, as well as recalling methods of contorting myself in ways I'm not sure I was meant to be contorted. While I didn't move the way I *used* to, I was back in action, leaping and spinning, twirling and gliding with a bit more delight than dexterity.

There came a day mid-fall when we were reintroduced to the art of the pirouette, the trademark turn of a ballerina. Let me start this by saying that, through my years of dance experience, I noted that there are *turners* and there are *jumpers*. I am a jumper. I have explosive strength and power, and could at one point probably leap the length of the stage in a single bound. I've always joked that my legs are nearly as wide as they are long, but rest assured that muscle mass this pronounced can make those babies *move*. I'm kind of like a classically trained bumblebee (in both stature and motion). The laws of physics suggest that bumblebees shouldn't be able to fly. But they do. Those same laws would probably suggest that I, too, shouldn't be able to fly. But I do. So, while I can soar like a bird with the best of them, my turns resemble confused ducks swimming in circles looking for stray bread crumbs on the surface of a pond. That being said, for most of my life I left the turning to fellow dancers more balance-prone than I.

The ballet mistress announced that we were to pirouette our way to the end of the room in a lovely combination of turns from the corner. I alternated between fear and dread as she demonstrated the routine. But, I recalled that my horoscope that morning indicated not only that I was "personality plus" that day but also that I would be "surprised at the results if I was willing to take risks." So, I took a deep breath, donned my best stage smile, and envisioned my flawless execution of the combination. And indeed, I was surprised.

With all the energy and hope I could muster, I started gliding across the diagonal of the room. The first was a tentative single turn. I not only completed it but it actually resembled a technically correct pirouette. A wave of relief moved through me. "I think I'll try a double," I coached myself. I glided through the preparation and nailed the double. "A double! Not bad. Maybe with age comes grace," I pondered. Next, I boldly attempted a triple and, much to my astonishment, "Praise, Hallelujah! I did it!" I proceeded to mentally congratulate myself with poor excuses for wordplay, like, "Maybe I've . . . hahaha . . . *turned* a corner with this skill." With a little giggle and a bit too much confidence, I figured, "Why not give it a *whirl* (hehehe) and try a quad?" And, with energy, gusto, and every good intention, I went through the now familiar preparation.

In my mind, I counted, "One . . . two . . . three . . . f . . ." The sentence was soon completed not with a *four* but with a four-letter word inappropriate to be included this book. Something had gone terribly awry. On hindsight, I'm thinking that I may have offended the bad-joke Gods that day, because what ensued was anything but a graceful display of balletic prowess.

Instead, it was like a really violent helicopter crash in a summer action-adventure blockbuster. First, the helicopter takes off and it looks like everything's going to be okay. The audience relaxes into the idea that these people are safe now, and they're reaching for their popcorn while they wait for the transition to the next scene. But suddenly, the popcorn goes flying because the copter's tail unexpectedly clips something—a burning building, a heat-seeking missile, the door of an alien warship—and starts to career wildly out of control. In painfully slow motion, it looks like a huge tetherball engulfed in flames, spinning on some imaginary axis toward the ground. The audio is heart-wrenchingly slow, too, with the *thud, thud, thud* of the copter's blades chopping the air behind the sound of the engine whining and screeching as it falls to earth. The camera shows another slow-mo close-up of someone yelling, "Noooooooooo . . ." and the helicopter finally crashes in an explosion of fire and mayhem and twisted wreckage. And then, silence. Onlookers are stunned. No one saw this coming.

And that's *exactly* what my quadruple pirouette looked like. I knew it from the moment my foot left the ground, as I felt myself tilting ever so slightly off balance. "Gravity is your friend," I stammered to myself. "Up*right*, not up*tight*!" But for all of my motivational platitudes, everything proceeded to go downhill from there. When the experience switched into slow motion in real time, I knew I was in *big* trouble. Not only had I overcorrected my balance, but I had used the tremendous strength in my "jumper's legs" to ensure I could make four revolutions. And, without a doubt, I *did* complete four revolutions. As a matter of fact, I think my total was more like seven or eight turns—a record for me. Of those seven or eight, two were completed nearly upright, one at a 45-degree angle from the ground, one almost parallel to the floor, and the others ended in a rather startling display of the previously described tumbleweed violently blown around the prairie by a tornado. In this case, I was the one who was shouting, "Noooooooooo . . ." in slow motion, but it was futile. The damage was done.

Through the ordeal, I proceeded to bruise, crack, and otherwise defile most of the bony parts of my otherwise well-padded anatomy. The room was deathly silent. You could hear a pin drop. And actually, I did, because the force of the impact actually blew my hairpins out of my bun and they lay strewn on the floor around me, minor debris from such a harrowing crash.

While onlookers thought I knocked myself out in the fall, I didn't. Instead, I experienced a brief dissociative moment, where I took a magic carpet ride to Aruba to determine if I could live there undiscovered for the rest of my life to avoid having to face anyone I knew after this incident. I was awakened from my reverie by the ballet mistress's matter-of-fact voice hovering over me, saying, "Well, you gave it a go, didn't you?" "Yes. Yes, I did," I replied. I gingerly scooped up the stray hairpins, along with the shattered remains of my dignity, and headed to the back of the room to try again—this time with just a touch more grace and a smidgen less centrifugal force.

A SLICE OF INSIGHT:
A DIFFERENT SPIN ON IT

Well, *that* sure hurt. Body. Mind. Ego. It was a spectacular display of gracelessness; a stunning show of sheer clumsiness. And yet, what I found was that even though my *body* didn't bounce as well as it used to, my *spirit* certainly did. In what I felt was a gutsy nod to the power of resilience, I headed right back there to try it all again. Well, maybe not *all* of it; maybe just the good parts. But I did, indeed go back, and I did it all again, *just a little bit differently than before*. I put a different spin on it in both body and mind.

But sometimes it can be hard to pick ourselves up after such a blow to our confidence (or our *competence*) and commit to starting again. In fact, it seems that it gets harder and harder as people age to throw caution to the wind in order to learn and grow unconstrained by fear. Children typically aren't inhibited by the fear of trying something new, which is why they so deftly learn to walk, talk, ride bikes, and scale jungle gyms. They know that their

> Children instinctively know that there are extraordinary benefits to be realized when you forgo your ego in favor of embracing your experience.

only job is to *try*, and that even though it may not work out perfectly the first, second, or even the fiftieth time, eventually it *will* work out because each time they make *just a little bit more progress*. And so they keep going. They tweak a little something after each attempt and gain a bit of strength with each try, and eventually they "bounce back" enough times that at some point they simply bounce to the next level of their development. Children instinctively know that there are extraordinary benefits to be realized when you *forgo* your *ego* in favor of *embracing* your *experience.*

But for some reason, as people age they tend to lose their perspective on this very basic principle of learning (and of living). And when they do, they tend to stay with the perceived *safety of the status quo* in lieu of exploring the *adventure of uncharted territory.* What we all need is a renewed commitment to welcome opportunities that *cultivate* both strength and flexibility rather than judging them as unpleasant or unfortunate *by-products* of living. In short, we need to relearn how to be resilient. When we embrace the power of resilience we create a much more meaningful (and memorable!) life experience. I refer to this as *mastering the art of the bounce.*

Resilience is our ability to "bounce back" from stress or challenges. It isn't born from safety or security, and it isn't cultivated from complacency or self-criticism. Instead, it's nurtured by taking reasonable risks and by trying out new ways of thinking and acting. It's fostered through equal parts challenge and creativity, practice and patience. The old adage, "If at first you don't succeed, try, try, again," is close but it really should read,

> **R**esilience is our ability to "bounce back" from stress or challenges. It isn't born from safety or security, and it isn't cultivated from complacency or self-criticism. Instead, it's nurtured by taking reasonable risks and by trying out new ways of thinking and acting. It's fostered through equal parts challenge and creativity, practice and patience.

"If at first you don't succeed, bring on the bounce, and try, try again."

So, for instance, when your attempt to text your son-in-law for the first time meets with the following phone message: "Deenie, typically when you use all capital letters in a text it implies that you are shouting, which I don't think you meant to do when you asked if I was feeling better and suggested I get some rest. Just checking, because it sounded kind of like a threat. But congrats on sending your first text," you have several ways of responding:

Potential response #1. Refuse to ever send another text to said son-in-law because you're too embarrassed you'll keep making errors and he'll keep a log of them, which he'll share at family gatherings as a form of cheap entertainment (which, incidentally, he probably *will* do).

Potential response #2. Call him and rephrase your text message in a motherly tone of voice on his voicemail, apologizing for not knowing the nuances of text messaging protocols, and assuring him that you have enrolled in an online course to remedy the situation, letting him know he'll receive texts from you sometime after you complete the curriculum.

Potential response #3. Send him the following text: "OIC. LOL. TYVM. HAGD." (Translated: "Oh, I see. Laugh out loud. Thank you very much. Have a good day," which you learn after a quick online search of texting shortcuts, and which he responds to with, "k btw TYCLO" (translated, "Okay, by the way, TURN YOUR CAPS LOCK OFF").

Yes, it's easier to bounce back (even *repeatedly*) when you do it *immediately*. So, when you knit your first scarf for someone and they ask how long it took your fourth-grader to complete it, knit one, purl two. And when your first attempt to install your new financial software requires three calls for tech support, program their number in your speed-dial if needed. Or, when your team leader suggests that your presentation to the rest of the staff "could have been a bit more polished," grab your nearest mentor and sit down to buff it

> **I**t's easier to bounce back (even *repeatedly*) when you do it *immediately* . . . resilience requires nothing more than the willingness to try again and the guts to act on something rather than just thinking about it.

up together. Resilience requires nothing more than the willingness to try again and the guts to *act* on something rather than just *thinking* about it (or worse yet, *lamenting* about it). When in doubt, keep taking another turn until you've achieved the results you're after!

MINDFULNESS BITE BY BITE: TURN, TURN AGAIN

1. Think of a recent stress or challenge in your life that took you off guard . . . something that you found difficult to "bounce back" from. (This could be a work disappointment, a disagreement with someone you love, or a goal you didn't quite reach.)

2. What could have enhanced your ability to bounce back? This could be anything: a shift in attitude, a little more time or patience, or some skill-training or support.

3. What one shift in thinking will help you "put a different spin" on setbacks in the future so you can "master the art of the bounce" and cultivate more resilience in this area of your life?

Fear of Flailing

I embarked on my first trip to the ski slopes at the ripe old age of twenty-six. I did so with a bit of trepidation given my complete lack of athletic ability and propensity for self-inflicted wounds of all sorts. Though, as you learned in the previous story, I was a classically trained dancer, I have found that I am typically prone to memorable feats of both insult and injury. In fact, my track record for self-inflicted wounds had become so solid that my husband was known to quip, "You're the only person I know who could hurt yourself on a donut." This was the standing joke in our household until it actually happened.

On the day in question, I helped myself to a donut hole from a batch of office goodies. I innocently tossed it to the side of my mouth and commenced my savoring protocol. By some mysterious force of nature, though, the renegade pastry lodged itself between my cheek and gum like a gigantic plug of chewing tobacco. Being an old-fashioned (and, as I later learned, a rather stale one), the donut's rugged surface proceeded to exfoliate the entire right side of my cheek when I extracted it. The abrasion was deep and painful enough that I actually abandoned the donut in favor of a saline flush. It was a *most* unsatisfying substitution.

I called my husband to share the bizarre turn of events. "Are you *serious*?" he asked. "You *literally* hurt yourself on a donut?

I don't even know what to say." I'm not sure that he was as shocked as he was concerned that he'd have to come up with some new way to describe my epic klutziness. My recent run-in with a blade-toting ciabatta, though, has offered him new ammunition.

The razor-sharp edge of said ciabatta sliced my upper lip with a surgeon's precision while I was enjoying my favorite roasted turkey and avocado sandwich at a local deli. Michael looked up from his meal to find me writhing in pain and bleeding out of the left side of my upper lip. "What *happened*? I look down for a *second* and when I look back up, you're *bleeding*. How did you manage *that*?" I relayed the turn of events, causing him to laugh until he choked on his club sandwich. Instant karma, if you ask me. "And I thought you couldn't top the donut incident but I was wrong. Only you, Deenie, only you." He was on the phone within minutes relaying "the ciabatta saga" to our grown daughters. In my defense, that ciabatta could have cut through a tin can and still slice a tomato with ease. It was the Ginsu of sandwich breads.

I share this with you to illustrate the fact that I can't even remain safe in the company of supposedly harmless baked goods, so we didn't really have high hopes for my prowess on the slopes. I had come to thoroughly appreciate the use of all of my limbs, so the notion of snapping one or more of them in the tradition of a turkey wishbone was unappealing at best. And yet, I tried to pump myself up for a good experience, thinking, "I can dance *Swan Lake*, damn it . . . How hard could it *possibly be* to stay upright on the bunny hill?" Evidently, it can be more difficult than I had imagined.

I donned my makeshift ski attire and headed up the mountain, where I first learned that *Swan Lake* and similar dance training had provided me with calves the size of a steroid-infused linebacker. And evidently, linebackers need special ski boots. After an hour of trying on nearly *every* piece of footwear in the place, a team of strapping young men harnessed me into a massive pair of what I can only describe as "man boots," and proceeded to manipulate themselves into a human version of vice grips to wedge me into them. The clasps strained against the pressure of my bulging calf muscles and I warned the other skiers to protect their eyes from flying metal fixings in the event these babies gave way. Somehow, though, the straps held and I hobbled up the mountain ready for action, despite knowing that these boots would no doubt—and very soon—sever my legs mid-shin. Honestly, I still have little divots there.

After a brief (and what I now recognize as highly ineffective) ski lesson, I was encouraged to make my way down the smallest bunny hill in the history of Nordic sports. I envisioned whooshing gracefully from side to side across the gentle slope of the hill, wind in my face, warm breath meeting cold air, one with nature. Then I would pop in a piece of Winterfresh gum, flash a radiant smile, offer an emphatic thumbs-up, and head in for some peppermint schnapps with a hot cocoa chaser.

Throughout my visualization exercise, it never even occurred to me that it would be beneficial to know which leg to put your weight on if you ever feel like turning. In hindsight, I realize that the ability to turn is a handy skill for successfully descending the slopes in one piece *with* control and *without* great disgrace. I realized this gap in my knowledge just as I reached the edge of the "skiable" part of the hill.

I quickly surmised that I had a 50/50 chance to choose the

correct leg and so, as I reached the turnaround point, I selected a leg at random and leaned into the turn. I promptly determined that I had opted for the wrong limb. I may have heard a game show buzzer faintly ringing in the background as I lurched haphazardly in the opposite direction of my planned turn, and a velvet-voiced announcer saying, "Oh, Johnny, *that* one's gonna hurt!"

I glanced at the ski lift above me, arms and legs thrashing as I headed out of bounds. I heard the first person calmly remark, "This isn't good" (which it wasn't). The second person nervously added, "She's out of control!" (which I was). And the third person anxiously belted out, "She's gonna hit that fence!" (which I did). Fortunately, the fence was one of those wobbly, forgiving structures that gently rebounded me into a perfect snow angel, limbs (but not ego) still intact.

I lay there for a while chuckling at my ability to career wildly out of control on a most decidedly un-careenable bunny hill. I then realized (after briefly grieving the loss of my dignity), that I had been given the chance to overcome my fear of flailing that day. Not *failing*, but *flailing*. I had *flailed* (and memorably, at that!), but I hadn't *failed*. I learned a valuable, unforgettable lesson about skiing basics while simultaneously providing riveting in-flight entertainment for those on the ski lift. Hey, the airlines charge six bucks for that!

A SLICE OF INSIGHT:
HAIL THE FLAIL

Perhaps my most important take away from this experience (other than thankfully intact bones and tendons), was that I realized that *the world had not stopped spinning because I hadn't*

*done something perfectly—or even well, for that matter—the
first time around.* In fact, the human race endured, my family
still loved me, and I was poised to ski better the next time. In
fact, on my very next attempt, I improved enough to avoid
eliciting running commentary from individuals on the ski lift.
Now that's progress. Although this run again proved that my
grace is more likely to be found on the *stage* rather than the
slopes, it was a markedly better attempt than my first.

> **E**ach time we stare *flailure* in the face, we get stronger and more confident in our ability to navigate new experiences and master what we deem worthwhile. When we release our fear of flailing, we learn faster and more effectively.

And so it goes in life, that each time we stare *flailure* in the face,
we get stronger and more confident in our ability to navigate new
experiences and master what we deem worthwhile. When we
release our fear of flailing, we learn faster and more effectively.
Wonky and wobbly at the start, those feelings quickly give way
to a sense of purpose and conviction honed by valiant efforts.

My clients and audience members often ask, "How can I get
over my fear of failure so I can move forward with my dreams?"
More often than not, what I find is that people are less fearful
of *failing* and more fearful of *flailing*. They are overwhelmed by
the prospect of looking stupid, feeling dumb, or allowing others to bear witness to their inevitable growing pains. So, they
often freeze up and do nothing. They panic at the thought of
trying something new, thinking they won't do it perfectly, or
they won't meet others' (or their own) expectations. They
worry that their imperfection will *repel* success instead of allowing them to *excel* at what they desire.

But, I'm suggesting that you'll be far better off when you embrace flailure. Everything worthwhile we've ever mastered we learned by flailing for a while until we got it right. When we learned to walk, talk, swim, or (let's be honest, now) even make love, we flailed around for a while until we built up our knowledge and skills, creativity, and confidence. Sure, there were false starts, some inevitable challenges, and a few comedic outtakes, but we focused on the *outcome* we wanted rather than the *manner* in which we were orchestrating it. So now, with all good fortune, we walk, talk, swim, and make love (amen to that) with a bit more certainty and a lot more intentionality.

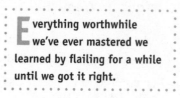

Everything worthwhile we've ever mastered we learned by flailing for a while until we got it right.

Why not "hail the flail" and see what new opportunities—and successes—might await you as a result? Hailing the flail simply requires making a *decision* to do something you're unsure of, an *appreciation* for how you'll benefit from the experiment, and a *support system* for giving it a go. Ultimately, with a little practice and a lot of patience, you'll learn the benefits of flailing with finesse.

MINDFULNESS BITE BY BITE: EMBRACING FLAILURE

1. What's one thing you have avoided doing because you were worried you would look stupid, disappoint yourself or others, or (gulp) *fail*?

2. How might you benefit from "hailing the *flail*" and giving it a try?

3. How will you make it easier on yourself to "embrace *flailure*" by enlisting support from other people or resources?

Out of the Mouths of Babes, Onto the Thighs of Women

I was attending one of my first big business trips flashing my shiny new public health degree, and I figured the hotel I had just entered must be the payback for all of those sleepless nights of churning out statistics problems and writing health promotion plans. In fact, like many of my readers, I probably could have written my thesis on the health impacts of consuming huge amounts of caffeine in order to finish a degree while working full-time. My resulting eye twitch finally subsided, and here I stood, at the incomparable Biltmore Hotel in Phoenix, Arizona, appropriately referred to as "The Jewel of the Desert." It's an icon of style and luxury bathed in the scent of massive vanilla candles adorning every console table in the place. Talk about opulence. This place had one of those cool life-sized chess games that you only see in old movies. I was starstruck by a rook of truly remarkable stature. The grounds were pristine, the rooms were elegant, and the pool was a glittering oasis. I credited all of those years of school for helping me quickly deduce that I probably could get used to this kind of life.

I was there with my good friend (and then-boss) Lyndia, to give a presentation at a national conference. Since we were public health professionals and good stewards of public dollars, we opted to share a room to save on costs (which was no big deal to me, since it turns out that this hotel room was the approximate size of my newlywed apartment back home). Lyndia had brought her son, Taylor, along, who was about three years old at the time, and we decided to hit the pool for a little rest and relaxation, as well as to implement our "toddler exhaustion initiative" to ensure we'd get a good night's sleep before the conference started.

We set about donning swimsuits and sunscreen, and took turns shuffling Taylor back and forth between us as we prepped for our day in the sun. Lyndia projected a rather unbecoming shade of green due to her uncontrollable morning sickness and I, with my Norwegian roots and proud Pacific Northwest pallor, displayed "a whiter shade of pale" that could effectively send SOS signals to low-flying airplanes in the event we were ever stranded in the desert. We made quite a striking pair.

I finished changing into my suit while she tasked herself with stocking the baby bag with enough juice to get through the afternoon and enough diapers to eventually collect the juice. I set about sunscreening Taylor and myself. It took all of fifty-seven seconds to coat Taylor thoroughly enough to allow him front-row access to the sun without having a single ray permeate his lily-white epidermis. As I had a bit more geography to cover, I began the lengthy process of slathering, twisting, and smoothing. At one point, I noticed Taylor standing in the corner in deep contemplation. "What's up, buddy?" I asked, warming myself up for some developmentally appropriate laps back and forth across the verbal pool. I waited for his answer, certain he was going to comment on how cool those little surfboards on his tiny swim trunks were or maybe he wanted to know what kind of floaties we would have access to at the pool.

Instead, he offered the following observation, in an objective but emphatic tone: "Your legs are WAYYYYYYYYYY bigger than my mom's." I blinked. Then I blinked again. I pondered, "How does one respond to a comment like that without inflicting bodily harm on an innocent three-year-old?" So I blinked some more. And thought about it.

I mean, sure, his mom is a tiny woman. So tiny, in fact, that even in her gloriously pregnant state, I could fit two of her in most of my wardrobe pieces. She's fortunate to have one of those enviable frames that allow her to shop in any store, wear any designer's line, and look stunning in any style, while others (myself included) roam seedier stores and dark aisles looking for old-lady textiles that scream, "Curve accommodating!" "Figure flattering!" and "Hidden tummy-slimming panel!" Would I forever be forced to don polyester/cotton blends that integrate far too much elastic into their designs? And yes, maybe I'd put on just a few (times two) pounds in grad school, and then in my days as a happy newlywed (and subsequently in my days as a disillusioned divorcee, but that's another story). But they wouldn't include pictures of me in tabloids with black bars superimposed on my eyes and a big "DON'T!" across my outfit? *Would* they?

All the while, Taylor is just looking at me inquisitively and nonjudgmentally. I stared back at him, still trying to figure out how to respond. Should I cry and run from the room? No. Primarily because there wasn't anywhere to go except for out into the foyer, and if a toddler thinks I look fat, chances are that random passersby might as well. My self-esteem couldn't take it. Should I just go ahead and admit that I've gained a bit of weight and query him about whether this swimsuit makes my butt look big? No. It just seems wrong to dump your body image issues on a three-year-old and then to expect reliable fashion advice from him. Should I pointedly reprimand him for violating one of the most revered of all etiquette rules and illustrate a Miss Manners lesson on the mirror using a bar of soap and a lipstick tube to sketch the silhouette of a plump woman next to one of those conversation bubbles, both in the middle of a huge, red circle with a slash through it? No, that could set him on the course toward sexist stereotypes and I'd no doubt get a call from Gloria Steinem one day scolding me for detracting from "the feminist cause."

So, instead I simply said, "Yes, everyone is a different size. That's what makes us human. Wouldn't it be *boring* if we all looked the same?" "Yeah," he replied, completely satisfied. And without any additional comments or queries, he padded off to chat it up with his mom. I sighed, stepped off the mental highdive that I planned on using to drown my self-esteem, and headed for the pool.

A SLICE OF INSIGHT:
BABIES DON'T GET TO DEFINE BABES

Isn't it amazing how we can undermine our self-concepts in a matter of seconds, without consciously *choosing* to, and without really *needing* to? When faced with an unexpected (and most times, *unintentional*) insensitive comment, we get sucked into a whirlpool of negative emotions, replaying the whole thing over and over in our minds, unwittingly collecting evidence that the comment is *true* rather than *trivial*. In this case, I was actually a healthy young woman with a relatively attrac-

> **W**hen faced with an unexpected (and most times, *unintentional*) insensitive comment, we get sucked into a whirlpool of negative emotions, replaying the whole thing over and over in our minds, unwittingly collecting evidence that the comment is *true* rather than *trivial*.

tive (though admittedly "shapely") physical stature. Overall, I felt pretty good about myself both fully clothed and in various stages of undress. All in all, I was doing fairly well for myself. And yet, within a matter of moments, I unconsciously allowed a toddler's innocent comment (which, as with all kids his age, was intended not as an *insult* but as an *observation*) to sabotage my self-image.

If you think about it, though, Taylor was just a convenient excuse for what I readily could have accomplished on my own accord (as could most women I know). We're masters of morphing what's *not* about us into something that *is* about us, even when it doesn't *serve* us. It's easy to look in the mirror (or at our work, or at our parenting, or at our home . . .) and unwittingly *magnify our shortcomings* instead of *celebrating our strengths*.

> **W**e're a society obsessed with focusing on our flaws instead of honoring our humanness. That just doesn't seem like the most satisfying approach to life.

We're a society obsessed with focusing on our flaws instead of honoring our humanness. That just doesn't seem like the most satisfying approach to life.

So, instead of complaining you have a big *ass* (sorry, Grandma!), maybe it's time to catalog your many *assets* instead. And, why not stop basing your *self-worth* on your *net worth*? Or, how about choosing not to judge yourself according to a *job title* and instead define yourself by *the*

*job you consistently do to make a difference in others' lives
(and in the world)*? In the end, only *you* get to define yourself,
your life, and your legacy on your own terms. And, just as I
learned, I hope you'll make the choice to stop allowing *babies*
to define who gets classified as a *babe*!

MINDFULNESS BITE BY BITE:
BE YOUR OWN BABE

1. Think about a few times when you've allowed someone
   (or something) else to impact how you felt about yourself.
   (Consider other people, the media, peers, or even items
   like your "skinny jeans.")

2. For each of those examples, how could you reframe your
   negative opinion into something *positive* (or at least more
   productive)?

3. In the future, what mantra will you use to remind yourself
   that you *always* have a choice about how you view yourself, regardless of how others view you? (Hmmm . . . why
   not "be your own babe"?)

CHAPTER 5

Resilience

From Sour to Sweet, the Transformation Is Complete

When Life Gives You Lemons, Make Lemon Meringue

A lot of people won't attempt to make lemon meringue pie because they think it's hard. There are more than a few steps involved and there are more than a few ways that the whole thing can go south. And then there are the people who can't imagine that *anything* as sour as a *lemon* could be transformed into something *sweet*. But oh, what they miss out on! Lemon meringue pie is kind of the "palate cleanser" of the dessert lineup. It wakes your taste buds up from their complacency with a bit of a shock followed by a smooth, pleasing finish. Your mouth and mind finally get it together and agree, "Yep, I'm alert now, I'm paying attention, and I'm thinking there's something altogether satisfying in this bizarre mix of flavors."

And, as you've come to expect by now, I believe that there's always some profound lesson to be learned from a pie. (It's not just a form of validating my vices, though that's certainly a part of it . . . I really believe that we learn most powerful concepts in some of the most unexpected places, including the pie plate.) The lesson here is that sometimes the experiences in life that feel the most shocking and sad and, thus, *sour*, can eventually yield something satisfying or *sweet* for us if we're open to that possibility, just like our faith in the lowly lemon can produce something as luscious as lemon meringue pie if we choose to use it that way.

So when challenges confront us—and they will with a frequency most of us don't really care for—we have the option of experiencing them, of feeling them, and of admitting that there's a real "punch" to them (or even a knockout on occasion). But at some point, we can find an element in the mix that brings us some relief. Or some peace. Or even some pleasure. It doesn't mean that we choose to ignore the fact that difficult things hurt, it's rather that we have the ability—if we stay aware and open—to realize that sometimes things in the least likely *packages* (like lemons) can yield an *outcome* (like lemon meringue pie) that opens our mouths or our minds in a new way.

The following stories focus on the situations in our lives where crises and chaos tend to ensue, but they also highlight the hope and healing that can be borne of those situations simply because they have *awakened* us. When we're alert we can experience so much more, whether it's in the form of awakened *senses*, which the pie can serve up, or awakened *appreciation* for the many things we have been blessed with in life, in spite of, and even emerging from, great hardship. This chapter illustrates that sometimes you can create something sweet out of something sour simply by being *open* to its possibility. We'll discuss the pie first, to offer you energy . . . and proof . . . that this can be done in the kitchen. Then we'll look at the stories of how this sour-to-sweet transition is possible *outside* of the kitchen.

Lemon Meringue Pie

Crust

Prepared pie crust for single 9-inch pie
½ cup graham cracker crumbs

Lemon Filling

1 cup sugar
¼ cup plus 1 tablespoon cornstarch
⅛ teaspoon salt
6 large egg yolks
1½ cups water
1 tablespoon lemon zest
½ cup fresh lemon juice (about 2–3 lemons)
2 tablespoons unsalted butter

Meringue

1 tablespoon cornstarch
⅓ cup water
¼ teaspoon cream of tartar
½ cup plus 1 tablespoon sugar
5 large egg whites
½ teaspoon vanilla extract

Preheat oven to 375 degrees.

Sprinkle pastry board with flour and ¼ cup graham crackers. Roll out pie crust into a circle. Sprinkle top of pie crust with flour and remaining ¼ cup graham crackers. Roll crumbs into top of crust. Place crust in 9-inch pie pan and flute the edges. Refrigerate for 30 minutes, prick with fork to avoid bubbling, and put in freezer for a few minutes.

Bake crust for 20–25 minutes until evenly brown (check several times to be sure it isn't bubbling). Set aside to cool.

Reduce oven temperature to 325 degrees.

Prepare lemon filling: Whisk sugar, cornstarch, and salt in a large, nonreactive saucepan. Stir in egg yolks and gradually whisk in water. Bring to a simmer over medium heat, and continue to cook for 8-10 minutes until thickened (whisk regularly). Remove pan from heat, whisk in lemon zest, lemon juice, and butter. Let cool slightly and transfer to cooled pie shell.

Prepare meringue: Combine cornstarch and water in a small saucepan. Bring to a simmer, whisking occasionally until thickened, and remove from heat when the mixture is thick and clear. Let stand until it is completely cold.

In a mixing bowl, mix cream of tartar and sugar. In a separate bowl, beat egg whites on high with a hand mixer until foamy. Add vanilla. Slowly beat in the sugar mixture 1 tablespoon at a time until stiff. Gradually beat in cornstarch mixture until stiff peaks form.

Spread meringue mixture over lemon mixture, starting at the edges and allowing to peak in the middle, swirling slightly and lifting with the back of the spoon as you go to form peaks.

Bake at 325 degrees for 15–20 minutes, until golden brown. Cool completely before serving.

Respiration, Not Desperation

We all have periods of time in our lives when it seems like everything that *can* go wrong, *does*. You never know when it's going to hit, but when it does, it hits without warning and it feels like being knocked out by a heavyweight prize fighter. For me, I call that time in my life "the soap opera years," because it involved an array of events that seemed not only *implausible* but nearly *impossible* to experience in the short span of only a few years. A back injury was followed by a layoff, which was followed by divorce, which yielded severe financial setbacks. These events were only interrupted by the unexpected deaths of both parents and my former husband. And then my cat died. I felt a little like an inhabitant of "Nietszche's Neverland" (referring to Frederick Nietszche's famous quote, "That which does not kill us makes us stronger"). Wow, did I do some power lifting during those years!

After dealing with the after*math* of these events for a number of years, I gradually started to be able to identify the after*laugh* associated with a few of them. That's when I knew the healing had begun. Now, in case it seems that I took *any* of these things lightly, let me assure you I did *not*. On the contrary, I know how just how heartbreaking they were for me (and are for others), but I also know what it took for me to feel *whole* and to find *hope* again. That's why I share some of these observations, because, since no one is immune to trauma or crisis or challenge in life, I believe that we can all benefit from learning about one another's healing journeys. And for me, the afterlaughs were critical turning points in my ability to live fully and love life again. The afterlaughs came after a significant investment of time, support, and processing, as well as a deeply personal and powerful relationship both with God *and* a really gifted therapist—now that's what I call a dream team!

Back to the story at hand. In my most evolved and philosophical interpretation of that epoch in my life, I can only sum up the experience in two expertly selected words, the likes of which literary types spend *years* trying to identify. *It SUCKED.* It sucked big-time. It sucked an everlasting gobstopper of grief and pain and heartache and devastation. No lie. But, after hearing that deafening, whooshing, sucking sound for what felt like an eternity, there came a moment of silence. And that silence ignited a tiny spark of insight that lit a candle of hope in my mind. You never really know *when* something like this will happen or *what* will bring it about, but you can identify it by the sigh of relief that finally passes your lips, often after a bout of unexpected and life-giving *laughter*.

Now, while I was fortunate to have been born with a very optimistic and resilient temperament, which can be downright handy during times like these, as you can imagine I was what concerned onlookers might describe as "a complete basket case" on and off throughout this period of my life. Upon reflection, I realize that I developed coping mechanisms that ranged from the benign (indulging in massive quantities of peanut butter–chocolate crispy treats for breakfast, lunch, and dinner for weeks at a time) to the balancing (acquiring various pieces of exercise equipment, perhaps in an effort to offset my considerable crispy consumption) to the bizarre (which involved the purchase of unnecessary cordless and/or cellular phones after each loss).

I eventually surmised that the phone-purchase trend was my

subconscious's way of suggesting that I might readily converse with dead relatives "on the other side" with my new turbo-charged Uniden 1.8 Ghz four-handset household communication system complete with caller id, three-way calling, answering machine, and free headset. Why so techno-riffic? I can only guess that because when one is communicating with individuals on alternate planes it might come in handy to chat hands-free while you're cooking dinner or weeding the garden, as well as to know who's calling, conference other family members in for a quick chat, and receive funny voicemails from loved ones in the sweet hereafter, including goofy rap songs on your birthday.

But honestly, the whole loss-a-rama started weighing heavily on me around trauma #6, and I started to feel the slightest bit sorry for myself. Okay, I'll come clean: It wasn't slight. It was a ginormous display of self-pity, the likes of which would raise the eyebrows of even the most accomplished teenage drama queen. My ability to bounce back had transformed from a sturdy rubber band into a cheap kickball left in the hot sun for too long. I was deflated and lifeless. I set about throwing myself a pity party of epic proportions. I surrounded myself with people who would validate the injustice of it all, who would hug me and shake their heads and bemoan with me the fact that "it's just not fair." I dabbled in both depression and happy hour (ah, the irony), and alternately wept silent tears and then became rigidly stoic, which would have been fine except I came across like a manic-depressive mime, and my husband can't *stand* mimes.

One day I found myself lamenting my fate with my mom, who was still there with me through trauma #6. She had been such a source of strength for me my whole life—my best teacher, my biggest advocate, and my most sincere supporter. She was the strongest and most compassionate person I've ever known. She was a great counselor and cheerleader, sometimes both in the same conversation. And, when necessary, she could also be an unapologetic realist with a flair for sharing succinct comments about life that you just don't necessarily *want* to hear but definitely *need* to. That often created an interesting dynamic.

On the day in question, I sat there in her living room recounting how *hard* everything had been and how *greatly* I'd suffered. She looked on with those warm, assuring eyes and just listened. I went on about how *wrong* it was, and how I really didn't know how much more I could *stand*. She nodded her head. I wrung out every last drop of emotional turmoil so she could help mop it up. And when I couldn't talk or cry anymore, I finished it up by blubbering, ". . . lost my dad, my health, my job, my husband (twice!), my credit rating, my cat. Honestly, the only thing I have left in the world is this little dog," and we both looked down at the saddest excuse for a pooch you could imagine.

He was a pudgy little mutt, lazy and apathetic, which garnered him the rather incongruous nickname "Sporto the nondog." His favorite pastime was staring at the wall like it was a movie screen, and he didn't take well to being interrupted. If you walked between him and the wall he'd look up in disdain, as if to say, "This, *rude woman*, is the best part. Get out of the *way*!" He also had a bad back, so if he took one wrong step as he descended the stairs (which were abundant in our home), he would catapult forward into a triple flip with a pike tuck before landing at the bottom of the stairway with a flourish, shaking and staggering his way into the living room. He had approximately four teeth left, which were in alternating locations in his mouth, making it rather entertaining to watch him attempt to gnaw his kibble. And his only talent was singing backup to Broadway show tunes with me. He simply had no dignity. And yet, he was the chubby, listless love of my life at that moment. How very apropos.

I closed my anguished plea for pity with that final sentence, "All I have left is this little dog," looked down at him, dabbed my eyes with the already soaked tissue in my hands, and shook my head. Then, I looked up at my mom and met her knowing eyes. I leaned in and waited for her sympathetic reassurance and sage advice, which I knew would change *everything* for me. And it most certainly did. She looked at the dog, looked at me, and simply said, "That dog . . . is *old*."

I had already started to relax my muscles in anticipation of her response, which I knew would be like a soft, warm blanket enfolding me in her compassion and wisdom. But when she uttered those words, I seized back up again. *"What?"* I said, thinking I hadn't heard her quite right. She repeated, plainly and with no emotion, "That dog . . . is *old*," continuing with, "He could die any day."

I raised my voice (a rare event in my mom's presence) and blurted, "Is that supposed to make me feel *better*, Mom? I'm sitting here waiting for you to tell me that everything is going to be okay and *that's* all you have to *say*? What the *hell* is *that* supposed to mean?" I recoiled on my own accord, prepared to be severely scolded like a teenager for swearing in addition to yelling at my mother. Instead of a stern admonishment, I received a succinct lesson in both psychology and philosophy that was far more effective than any of my college courses.

"Well," she said, as matter-of-factly as she could, "if you're resting your happiness and hope for the future on that sorry excuse for a dog, you've got a lot bigger problems than what you've gone through so far. That dog could die any day, and *then* what are you going to do?"

I was shocked. And aghast. And then I was duly offended on behalf of my snuggledy-buggledy love dog. I looked down at him, prepared to give her a piece of my mind (though admittedly there wasn't much left to give), and realized that she was absolutely *right*.

A SLICE OF INSIGHT: TO BREATHE AND TO BENEFIT

While I don't recall her *exact* words after that (which I'm sure commenced with some version of, "Don't you raise your voice at me, young lady," followed by a cascade of astute observations about my current situation), upon reflection I finally distilled the *essence* of what I believe she was trying to get across to me. It goes a little something like this: "You'd better think about how you want to move forward from all this, because there will *always* be something else that will knock the wind out of you. You have the ability—the privilege, in fact—to stop, take a deep breath, and *choose* your future with pur-

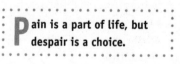

Pain is a part of life, but despair is a choice.

pose instead of just *complaining* about your past or present. *Pain is a part of life, but despair is a choice.*"

Her unanticipated candor that day helped me learn how to make *conscious* decisions about the *meaning* I give to unpleasant situations and what I want to *do* as a result of that meaning. And that's when I uncovered the real significance of her suggestion (to stop, take a deep breath, and choose your course of action). Maybe we're called to live our lives through a process of *respiration*, rather than *desperation*.

> **M**aybe we're called to live our lives through a process of *respiration*, rather than *desperation*.

So much of our response to the unpleasant and unexpected is reactionary and fear-based, and for good reason—these things can be incredibly uncomfortable and we want those negative emotions to go away, and to *go away fast*. So, we breathlessly take quick action (often in the wrong direction) to stave off feeling bad. Whether it's through denial or distraction, substances or self-pity, we often mask an emotion in the short term to avoid the discomfort associated with it. But over the long haul, that's a rather unproductive approach that often yields more *hardship* than *relief*.

> **M**ost of the challenges we face today (even the worst of them) are not *physical* incidents that threaten our very lives, but rather *emotional* experiences that threaten our opportunity to truly *live*. The difference in our response is dependent on whether we choose to *survive* or to *thrive*.

It's a fact that our bodies and brains respond to threats with *lots* of adrenaline and very *little* conscious thought. We go into an auto-pilot mode that was genetically designed to help us *survive* when faced with threat to life or limb. And yet, most of the challenges we face today (even the worst of them), are not *physical* incidents that threaten our very *lives*, but rather *emotional* experiences that threaten our opportunity to truly *live*. Our response differs based on whether we choose to *survive* or to *thrive*. To me, the latter is the obvious choice.

Research proves that your breath can be used as the "reset" button for both your mind and your body. As my good friend Bob Maurer (author of *One Small Step Can Change Your Life*) says, "Your breath is the accelerator pedal for stress." In the time it takes to fill your *lungs* with life-giving *air*, you can consciously

> **Y**ou'll not only have a reason to *live*, but to live *fully* and *vibrantly* and well when you choose *respiration*, rather than *desperation*.

choose to fill your *mind* with life-giving *thoughts*. That choice comes from purposefully deciding to change your perspective, survey your options for next steps, and decide how you want to write the next chapter in your life, even if you didn't much care for the last one. Thus, even if your dog is old (and could kick the bucket any minute now) or you're faced with some other unfortunate circumstance in your own life, you'll not only have a reason to *live*, but to live *fully* and *vibrantly* and *well* when you choose *respiration*, rather than *desperation*. That's all it takes. Just one full, deep, healing, soothing, future-shaping breath at a time.

MINDFULNESS BITE BY BITE:
INHALE FOR INSIGHT

1. In what areas of your life or incidents in your past have you allowed yourself to be the perpetual guest at a never-ending pity party?

2. Identify a particular situation in your life that could benefit from focusing on *inhaling* as you seek insight, ideas,

inspiration, or the initiative to help you create a more favorable outcome for yourself.

3. How can you remind yourself in the future to focus on *respiration* rather than *desperation*?

A Real Undertaking

I have to say that, strangely, some of the most memorable times that laughter has changed my life for the better were during times of grief. It's true, some people are offended at the notion of laughing during times of hardship or loss, but I'm a firm believer that laughter, when dispensed with care and compassion, can provide hope and healing like nothing else. It can be an incomparable remedy for body, mind, and soul. I learned that lesson at age twenty-four, when I lost my father unexpectedly to a heart attack.

Dad was only fifty-nine, and this was the first truly traumatic experience I endured in life. Yes, the loss of a parent is one of those inevitable loop-de-loops we experience as we travel round the circle of life. (Thank you, Elton John and *The Lion King* for imbedding that score into readers' minds for the rest of the day.) But the stoic observation that loss is "just part of life" doesn't begin to staunch the flow of sorrow from grief-imposed wounds. Sometimes you have to slog through the muck for a while until you eventually find comfort in a memory, or an insight, or (with luck) a laugh.

Dad's death was a blow to all of us, as he was a remarkable man with a quick wit, infectious laugh, extraordinary intellect, and loving nature. Fortunately, I am blessed (many times over,

I might add) to have a large, cohesive, and almost alarmingly loving family. Along with my stepmother, Kay; my eight sisters and brothers (full, half-, and step-, a true modern family); and their respective partners, we set about planning the service to pay tribute to an unforgettable man.

We were all devastated, overwhelmed, and filled with dread about the prospect of moving forward in this world without a dad to call when we had a question about European history or when we wanted the best strategy for preparing ginger steak with just the right panache. (Sometimes, unbidden, we'd get the history lesson *along* with the ginger steak recipe, thus my familiarity with the role of the spice trade among European explorers, including the historical fact that at one time saffron was more valuable than gold. Add that little tidbit to your tavern trivia night tool belt.)

Now that Dad was gone, how would we perfect our respective pool games? (In fact, I never actually did, with the dubious distinction of leapfrogging more balls off the table onto the feet of passersby than into the pockets of the pool table.) How would we ever learn the nuances of effective, though gratuitous, dog training? (It's infinitely more amusing than productive to teach a dog to play dead when someone points a finger at her and says, "Bang!" and yet it still takes remarkable skill and patience.) Who would we call when our car engine catches fire, even prior to calling the fire department (kids, don't try this at home) or when we needed a synonym for a term paper at midnight (don't expect a perky voice, but do expect the perfect word)? These were the unanswered questions we pondered as we sat there at the funeral home listening off and on to the funeral director plan the service.

We were all weeping uncontrollably—all nineteen of us—and simply handed the tissue box from person to person like a collection plate at church, where you accept it, nod slightly, offer a modest attempt at a smile, and hand it to the next person. We cycled through our grief like the wave at a baseball game—you could see the contagion move through the room and then settle down at the other side, only to return again with seamless transition from person to person. Our sadness felt like a heavy wool blanket in that hot room—unwanted, uncomfortable, and overwhelmingly unpleasant. And then something happened that changed it all for me . . . at least for a few precious moments.

The funeral director had completed most of the planning for the service, and then queried us on whether we'd like to arrange for an escorted processional to the cemetery. He began explaining the benefits and drawbacks of the process, noting that, "On one hand, it keeps people together and keeps the services timely, which is a plus with a family as large as yours. On the other hand," he continued, "it requires hiring staff and cars to ensure that traffic stops along the way for safety and efficiency. It's a significant addition to the cost, which is yet another consideration." We all looked at each other blankly, as nothing was really registering by this time. He realized that we had just about reached our threshold for both planning and grieving that day, so the funeral director attempted to bring the matter to a close with one final suggestion. "While I like to recommend using the processional, I understand that, due to cost and scheduling, it really can be quite an *undertaking*."

I stopped mid-whimper and cocked my head like a confused dog. "Did he just say what I *think* he said?" I asked myself.

"Did an *undertaker* really just use the word *undertaking*?" That was followed by the obvious next question, for which I had no answer, "Is this some kind of *funeral home humor*? I started to snicker, so I looked down and tried to stifle it. I didn't want to be forever deemed the inappropriate one *here* of all places (because inevitably I'm the one deemed inappropriate in all *other* places). But, the psyche can only bear so much distress in one day before eventually it just gives up. And that's what happened. My snicker turned into a giggle and the giggle turned into a chuckle and the chuckle turned into a laugh and then I was, please forgive the pun, a *complete goner*.

My laughter was uncontrollable, coming in irrepressible swells. Tears of grief were soon (and gratefully) replaced by tears of laughter, which became even more pronounced as I repeatedly tried to remind myself that *this is simply not the time nor the place when one is supposed to laugh*. But none of my siblings had caught the unfortunate play on words, so I was left to writhe around snickering like I'd gone mad while several of them pondered a short trip up the hill to admit me into the psychiatric unit of the local hospital.

What I experienced that day was one of the most powerful feelings of *release* and, thankfully, *relief* that I've ever felt. Most of the time we find ourselves drowning in grief, thrown around in waves of devastation like we're being tossed about on white-water rapids of loss. We can barely breathe, and we most certainly can't determine which way is up. It feels like we keep getting sucked under, only to gasp for breath every now and then. Periodically, someone extends a compassionate hand in a rescue attempt, but sometimes the current is too strong and we continue to be pulled under.

But then, as unexpectedly as those raging waves take us under and toss us to and fro, we suddenly see above us a limb that we reach out and grasp, and we cling to it for safety and respite from that river. As we sit there gasping for breath, trying to gain our bearings, we realize that we're closer to shore than we thought and that, even though the swim there might *feel* impossible given our sheer exhaustion, we suddenly recognize we can save ourselves. That moment of rest, the safety of that limb, is sometimes an unexpected but desperately needed moment of *laughter*. That's what it was for me in that moment. Although no one else shared that feeling of relief with me, it provided me with just enough of a buffer from my pain to know that I *could* and eventually *would* laugh again. That this was just the beginning of my healing. And when I finally calmed down enough to share the story with some of my siblings, *they* laughed, too. So *I* had the honor of being the branch that rescued *them* from the rapids that day, as well. And what a gift that was—to pass on the healing power of laughter to someone else in need at just the right moment.

A SLICE OF INSIGHT:
THE REAL WAY TO HEAL

I find it fascinating that when I share a variety of stories in my speeches and shows, it's often the ones about challenges and hardship, grief and loss that spark the most comments from the audience. Inevitably people seek me out to thank me for exploring the notion that there's no magic time line or process for grieving and going on. Everyone has different ways of healing

and everyone is entitled to experience their own pain in their own
way, including through both
laughter and tears. There's no *right*
way to heal—there's only *your* way of healing.

> **T**here's no *right* way to heal—there's only *your* way of healing.

But this idea of navigating challenges in your own way isn't confined to dealing with the loss of a life. It's equally important to follow your unique path after the loss of a job, a relationship, a long-held goal, or even your health. It seems that we tend to believe the mistaken notion that *serious things always demand serious responses*. While *often* they do merit a sober tone, they don't *always*. Difficult situations can sometimes beckon us to share our *humanity* with the world, complete with its stunning array of imperfections and vivid display of unique responses to tough times. Which certainly can include laughter, among other things.

> **D**ifficult situations can sometimes beckon us to share our *humanity* with the world, complete with its stunning array of imperfections and vivid display of unique responses to tough times.

I truly believe that there are times (only when you're ready) when one of the greatest healing gifts you can give yourself is either to laugh until you cry, or to cry until you laugh. Or both. I shared this notion with a fellow attendee at the Hawaiian Islands Writers Conference. She was a native Hawaiian who had a warmth and peace about her that helped me feel instantly at ease. We felt an immediate connection. I shared some of the concepts from this book and my one-woman show based on it, and she nodded in appreciation. We talked about this notion that sometimes people take exception to the idea of laughing when you *should* be crying, and then mutually wondered, "Who gets the privilege of defining that *should*, anyway?"

My wonderful new friend offered what I thought was an outstanding spin on the idea of laughing until you cry or crying until you laugh. She noted that we view our life and its inevitable ups and downs in ways that are influenced both by our cultural backgrounds and by our personal life experiences, among other things.

> Even in the most difficult of "undertakings," we do, indeed, deserve the chance to laugh until we sigh.

She offered the following: "In Hawaii, we live the spirit of Aloha, which means, among other things, 'the presence of breath' or 'the breath of life.' As you were speaking, it dawned on me that one of my most treasured feelings is when I've laughed so hard that I experience a sense of release, which then gives way to a profound feeling of peace. So, for me, rather than only crying until we laugh, or laughing until we cry, don't you think that sometimes in situations like these, what we really want to do is laugh until we *sigh*?" It made such sense to me. Regardless of our chosen process for moving through life itself, or through the pain and loss it sometimes brings, don't we all deserve the opportunity to feel that sense of relief . . . of release . . . of peace? Even in the most difficult of "undertakings," we do, indeed, deserve the chance to *laugh until we sigh*.

MINDFULNESS BITE BY BITE: CRY WAY, SIGH WAY, MY WAY

1. Identify a circumstance that has brought about pain or grief, fear or uncertainty that you don't feel you have

fully healed from. (This can be something small or something big.)

2. What elements of that experience speak to you—can you identify something you learned, something that changed you in a meaningful way, or an aspect that was worthy of either a healing laugh, cry, or sigh (or some other form of release)?

3. What can you do to give yourself "permission" in the future to experience—and to heal from—challenge and loss in your life *in your own way* rather than thinking there is a *right* way?

Dr. Uptalker

Life often sends us an eclectic mix of tragedy and comedy just to wake us up. This tale is just one example of that Shakesperean shake-up. My mother was quite ill on and off for about a decade, and my sisters and I spent a good part of our teen and young adult years making ourselves comfortable in a most diverse array of hospital, physician, clinic, and pharmacy waiting areas.

From those experiences, we could list the cafeteria menus and daily specials by memory (food fosters the transition between distraught and distraction) and rated each experience based on the quality of waiting room reading material, convenient rest room access, and the tolerance of the nursing staff with regard to our sometimes rather overcaring (or is it overbearing?) personalities. We divvied up our waiting times by tag-teaming the completion of thousand-piece "serene meadow landscape" puzzles while expertly deflecting the attempts of stray children to scale life-size statues of Jesus in our local Catholic hospital.

We took turns doing schoolwork, needlework, or social work in the company of other medical-center regulars and learned the very best positions for lulling oneself to sleep in upright chairs and on lumpy couches, while balancing stray body parts on gurneys, or strewn two-to-a cot in my mother's room. To this day, though most people are fearful of hospitals, I feel a strange sense of calm when I walk through those doors, not only because my mom was a nurse for thirty-five years, but also because I spent a good portion of my developmental years bonding with family and friends amid monitors and medical supplies. Okay, maybe it's just a *bit* peculiar but I find the smell of disinfectant strangely comforting, even though it can never be found in my own home.

During this particular hospital stay, my mother's health had declined rather significantly and rapidly. She suffered many ailments, with most of her body systems on sabbatical after a lengthy tenure of overwork, so it was quite a task to keep up with the medication regimens and treatment protocols for kidneys, veins, heart, and lungs, not to mention the various procedures for cancer, diabetes, and, during this stay, matching broken ankles.

Given all of the maladies, it was becoming increasingly more like a game show in her room every day, with new contestants and questions and prize packages. I'd imagine each doctor initiating our consult with a *Jeopardy!*-type statement such as, "The appropriate schedule for dialysis this week," and we were supposed to say, "What is three times a week or Monday/

Wednesday/Friday?" "Correct," he would say, and we'd move on to Double Jeopardy!, where we had to wager some percentage of our stash of Junior Mints based on our knowledge of "The Electrifying Endocrine System."

Or we'd get into a *Price Is Right*–type conversation, where we'd be bidding on her estimated discharge date and one of my sisters would say, "Well, Bob, I'm going to bid nine days," followed by "I'll bid eight," and "I'll go for five." Whomever wanted to manipulate the situation (yes, typically me) would say, "I'll bid *one* day, Bob," and we'd hear Johnny's voice announce, "That's right, Bob! Deanna was the closest to the projected discharge date of four days without going over. Deanna, you just won a *brand-new wheelchair and a matching walker* for your mom!" And there would be applause and high-fives and the uttering of "Oh my gosh . . . I can't believe I really won!"

On the day in question, her health had declined to such an extent that everyone was having trouble keeping up with the various treatment protocols and providers (including the providers themselves). As such, we requested a meeting with all of the physicians and the head nurse to learn how they were working together to address my mother's needs. There we sat in the conference room, fueled by equal doses of anxiety and caffeine. It was obvious she wasn't doing well, but we were all trying to act like it wasn't as serious as it was, masking our rising panic at the thought that this might very well *not* turn out well. We were polite and welcoming to all of the doctors, grateful they had made time for this healthcare huddle on such short notice. Everyone went around the room introducing themselves and, as I listened to the array of expertise in the room, I was stunned. The collective amount of education and years of medical experience could have probably found a cure for cancer that day, but their sole focus in that moment was on Mom. What a blessing.

They introduced themselves one by one: the heart doctor, kidney doctor, internal medicine specialist, vein doctor, cancer specialist, lung doctor, bone doctor, and on and on. It was an alphabet soup of anatomy and an orchestra of vital organs. About halfway through the parade, I figured we'd eventually be meeting every doctor in the history of American pop culture. After Dr. Smith, Dr. Jones, and Dr. Johnson, I thought, "Wait a minute . . . did he just say Dr. *Seuss*?" Oh yeah, and there's Dr. Spock, Dr. Dolittle, Dr Pepper, Dr. Zhivago, and Dr. Dre. Farther down the room, you'll see Doc Martin, Doc Holliday, and Doc from the Seven Dwarfs (who nods his head and shares a cordial, "Hi ho!"). And rounding the table (and the end of our list), Trapper John, MD, and Marcus Welby, MD.

I tried to refocus, but it was no use, because by then it started to feel a tad bit like a twisted *Dr. America Pageant*. "Hello, I'm Dr. Jones. I hail from Baylor College of Medicine (applause). In my free time, I love to perform interpretive splenectomies and practice suturing blindfolded with one hand tied behind my back while riding a unicycle. If I had one wish for humanity it would be that every person would live their life with the precision of a surgical incision—clean, straight, and prone to minimal scarring." And then the next provider would step up to the microphone. Refreshed by my mental television break, I reminded myself that the purpose of our meeting was critical to all of us—we wanted the very best coordinated care for my mom—so I forced myself to listen, though I have to admit that

I secretly expected one of the docs to digress into a baton twirling routine.

I reoriented myself to the task at hand and stayed engaged for most of the meeting. Near the end of our time together, one final physician chimed in to sum up the course of treatment. He was handsome and self-assured, and you could tell he was ready for this meeting to be over with, so he guided us toward closure. He started with, "Let me summarize what I think we heard today from all of the physicians and the family," and we listened intently. His one-way conversation went something like this:

"Is your mother a very sick woman? *Yes*, she *is*.

"Do we think she's going to die today? *No*, we *don't*.

"Is it going to take a hell of a lot of coordination between the providers to bring her the very best healthcare outcomes? I think we all *agree* to *that*.

"Will she need a good team of people supporting her rehabilitation and recovery? You *bet* she *will*.

"Are we all committed to making sure that happens? *Yes*, this meeting *proves* it."

And it went on. And on. And on. Every single aspect of his summary was posed as a question, which he proceeded to answer himself. I tried not to laugh. Sincerely, truly, madly, deeply, honestly, I did. I held it until I nearly passed out from the side-splitting pain of holding it in. But he just kept coming up with them. It felt like we had landed right in the middle of a Seinfeld episode called "Dr. Uptalker."

I looked around the room at my sisters, like usual, wondering, "Is anyone else *getting this*? Or is it just *me*?" (Which, quite frankly, I frequently find is indeed the case.) No one else had picked up on it. So I had to resort to my own devices to get through it. I found myself coming up with various additions to his dialogue, secretly suggesting lines such as:

"Do you sound like a complete idiot? *Yes*, you *do*.

"Is there any reason I should take you seriously right now? *No*, I don't *think* so.

"Will I burst a critical artery soon if I hold this laughter in much longer? *Yes*, I'm sure I *will*."

I glanced around for an out, but I didn't want it to appear that I wasn't taking the situation seriously (which in that moment, I can honestly say I wasn't). So I harnessed the most spectacular display of willpower I have ever mustered, knowing it wouldn't be long until the meeting ended. I held it in. And it hurt. Badly. My stomach started to convulse and my shoulders started to heave. I looked down at the table and let my hair fall into my face so no one could see I was laughing. As I gently shook from laughter, one of my sisters (to this day I'm not sure which one) patted me on the back to soothe my "crying" and assure me that it would all be okay. Just as I thought I'd give myself a stroke from the pressure of holding it in (confident that I'd receive great care from the physicians in that room if that did happen), the meeting ended and I was able to mutter "Thank you" to all of the providers as they left the room.

And then I laughed until I cried. And cried for a while longer—that kind of cry that allows *fear* to give way to *freedom* (if only for a few moments). And then, thankfully, once again I cried until I laughed. It was a little dose of mental morphine that briefly dulled the unbearable pain of witnessing the suffering of someone you love so dearly.

When all was said and done that day, I heard Dr. Uptalker's voice in the recesses of my mind asking, "Will this laughter help you feel better *forever*? *No*, probably *not*. Will it help you feel better in *this* moment, even if there aren't many others to be had right now? Why, *yes*, yes, it *will*." And that, my friends, was good medicine.

A SLICE OF INSIGHT:
A PRESCRIPTION FOR POSSIBILITIES

It's no crime to insert a bit of silliness into the seriousness of life. It doesn't minimize or trivialize your experience to find small things that provide a dose of respite during the most difficult times. Laughter during times of sadness is as appropriate as any other way of expressing emotion, provided it doesn't infringe on others' experience in a disrespectful way. We each have a unique way of healing from life's inevitable hardships.

And sometimes, humor can be a soothing balm on the painful wound that fear or loss creates. During times of crisis, while laughter doesn't *cure* what ails us, it certainly can *calm* our nerves and *channel* our energy toward more productive ways of thinking.

> **D**uring times of crisis, while laughter doesn't *cure* what ails us, it certainly can *calm* our nerves and *channel* our energy toward more productive ways of thinking.

When I experienced hardship growing up, I recall my parents saying so many times, "This, too, shall pass." It's an almost universal way of offering the comfort that only hope can provide during the worst of times. I find myself saying the same thing to my children, whether talking with Amber about the challenges of parenting, Rhiannon about health issues, or Malina about school bus insults. The topics vary, but the message is often the same. As I've done some reflecting on this statement, though, I've wondered just *how* these things finally "pass"?

Is the whole "time heals all wounds" notion part of the equation? Well, certainly time can *dull* pain and *define* new experiences to offset the old, but I don't think it actually *heals* all wounds. Is it love, which "bears all things," that enables us to go on? It sure *helps*—after all, love is the great *unifier* and, at times like these, it can also be the great *pacifier*. But it doesn't *erase* hardship . . . it simply *eases* it. Is it *compassion* that does the trick? Well, it certainly can't hurt, because, as the Dalai Lama says, "If you want *others* to be happy, practice compassion. If *you* want to be happy, practice compassion." But compassion is only one element that helps us *endure* something difficult as we work toward *embracing* a new reality. Or, is it *laughter*, which has forever been referred to as "the best medicine"? Maybe it's not the *cure-all*, but it certainly makes the condition more *bearable*.

Whether you are grieving the loss of a job or a relationship, an opportunity or a person, how can you set the stage for "This, too, shall pass"? If you sense *time* will help you heal, perhaps you can allow yourself a generous time line to recover from setbacks without thinking you're taking *too long* or questioning whether you're taking *long enough*. Or, maybe you can gift yourself with periodic diversions (whether it's a good book or a good meal) that take your mind off of disappointment, if only for a short while. If you think *love* will help you recover from a challenge, why not surround yourself with people who care about you and ask for their support without fear of burdening them? Or, choose to shower others with your affection and appreciation (a show of love that benefits both of you)?

If it's *compassion* you need, why not begin by showing *yourself* compassion through the knowledge that there are no rules for recovering from crises, and that you aren't required to *think* or *act* or *be* a certain way to get through this situation? Or consider showing compassion to someone else in need by extending a smile, a hug, or a helping hand. If it's *laughter* that you think will mend your heart or restore your hope, *first* give yourself *permission* to laugh, and *then* consider *sharing* a funny insight with a friend or family member. And, when needed, ask your loved ones to help *you* find humor when you're having trouble seeing it on your *own*.

> When we want to maintain the hope that "This, too, shall pass," it seems like this prescription of time, love, compassion, and laughter might just do the trick.

So, when we want to maintain the hope that "This, too, shall pass," it seems like this prescription of time, love, compassion, and laughter might just do the trick. And if that prescription is administered on occasion by someone like Dr. Uptalker, all the better. "Are there rules or time lines for healing 'correctly'? No, there aren't." "Do we have a choice about how to heal on our own terms and in our own ways? You bet we do." It's time to exercise that choice. There's no need for a consult or a care plan, just a bit of reflection and a personal decision. And perhaps even a moment of laughter.

MINDFULNESS BITE BY BITE:
HOPE, HEALING, AND HUMOR

1. Think of a circumstance in your life when you were stressed, anxious, fearful, or sad (or, as is often the case, all four at once).

2. When you reflect on that time, can you identify anything that occurred that could have lightened your experience even the tiniest bit? Is there something you didn't notice (or didn't feel comfortable enough to acknowledge) that might have provided a sense of *hope* that "This, too, shall pass"?

3. Since challenging times are a universal experience, how might you prepare your mind *now* to be open (without judgment) to aspects of difficult experiences in the future that could provide hope, healing, or even humor?

CHAPTER 6

Release

The Meltdown Makes Miracles

Melting for Maximum Benefit

Sometimes it takes a meltdown to create a new and improved situation that better suits us than the existing one. I always remember this as the concept of "recasting," which I was first introduced to in a great book called *How We Choose to Be Happy*, by Rick Foster and Greg Hicks. In metalwork, the process of recasting involves melting down metal in order to create something new, like a work of art or useful tool. The imagery has always been profoundly memorable to me, and it's always been a reassuring reminder of the fact that when we *release* something from one form (whether that thing is a habitual way of thinking, a relationship, a goal, or anything else), we can often *create* something even more pleasant or practical in a new form. After the meltdown comes the magic.

That's why I chose chocolate meltdown pie to reflect this important truth. This pie is one of the *easiest* and, at the same time, exquisitely *decadent* desserts you can enjoy, and it all comes from melting down the original form of the chocolate, blending it with things that enhance it, and recasting it into a brand-new work of chocolate art. Who needs Michelangelo when you can create an artistic rendering of universal truths through the medium of 65 percent cacao? Sign me up for that kind of art class!

Chocolate aside, often in life we stay attached to the status quo (sometimes consciously, sometimes not), because it's easier or more comfortable for us than deciding to do things differently. So, even if our current situation is *less* than fulfilling or *more* than frustrating, we tend to keep things as they are to avoid the meltdown that we assume will be too painful or too messy or too unmanageable. And sometimes, even when our current experience is *good*, we stay right where we are instead of letting go of what we know in order to experience something *great*.

This chapter focuses on this concept of *releasing*—on the idea that sometimes we create both more *space* and more *possibility* in our lives when we let go of something we *know* in order to make room for ourselves to *grow*. The stories are about recognizing the need for change, and about taking risks and making choices that move us forward rather than holding us back. But first, to illustrate that meltdowns can create miracles, we'll start with the chocolate meltdown pie recipe and then move on to examine how those times in our lives that feel like meltdowns can produce miracles of their own.

Chocolate Meltdown Pie

2 large eggs
½ cup plus 1 tablespoon all-purpose flour
½ cup granulated sugar
½ cup packed brown sugar
¾ cup (1½ sticks) softened butter
1½ cups chocolate chips
1 cup chopped walnuts, pecans, or macadamia nuts
1 unbaked 9-inch deep-dish pie shell
Vanilla ice cream or whipped cream, optional

Line oven with foil or "drip catcher," or have a baking sheet handy to catch drips from the baking pie. Preheat oven to 325 degrees.

In a bowl, beat eggs on high speed until foamy. Mix in flour, granulated sugar, and brown sugar. Beat in butter. Stir in chocolate chips and nuts. Pour into pie shell.

Bake 55–60 minutes or until knife inserted in center of pie comes out clean. Cool for at least 15 minutes.

Serve warm with ice cream or whipped cream, if desired, and marvel at the miracle that a meltdown can produce!

The Blue Flip-Flop

It was nearing the end of a very long winter, with the germ warfare it wages on snowbound families at an all-time high. My son, Carsten, six months old at the time, had started spiking a wicked fever early one Saturday. Michael and I were floating his limp little body in a lukewarm bath, alternately soothing him and ourselves, and cataloguing our weekend medical provider options while our five-year-old daughter, Malina, and her nine-year-old cousin, Jacob, entertained themselves in the family room. It had been eerily quiet for some time, and as most people know, young children and unexpected silence are never a good pairing. In the midst of caring for Carsten, it never really dawned on me that this was the calm before the storm.

Suddenly, Malina came barreling into the bathroom, cupping her hand over her nose. She was bleeding profusely and her eyes were darting around like a trapped animal. I leapt to my feet and said, "Malina . . . what happened?" Through the faucet pouring out of her nose, she stammered, "I got a flip-flop up my nose!" I immediately pictured the typical outcome of children's horseplay gone awry, with Malina as the recipient of a well-executed (though poorly planned) kick in the face—not such an uncommon experience with kids of their age. And then it dawned on me. With several feet of snow blanketing our home, flip-flops were neither *acceptable* attire nor, I might add, *accessible* to her in the dead of winter.

"Malina," I posed, "what do you *mean* you got a flip-flop up your *nose*? Your flip-flops are in the bin of summer clothes." (In retrospect, it seems this clarifier may have been unnecessary mid-crisis. Hindsight suggests that there might be a more appropriate time to discuss protocols for organizing off-season clothing, perhaps one that did not involve the imminent loss of consciousness due to low blood volume.)

Due to the swelling in her nose, her response came in the form of a language that resembled English, but that replaced the "m" in every sentence with a "b," and every "n" and "t" with a "d." She had nailed a perfect cartoon character voice, replete with sarcasm and disgust, though we couldn't fully appreciate it due to the gravity of the situation. It resulted in the following communication: "Do, *BOB*, I got a flip-flop up by *DOZE*. A Polly Pocked flip-flop *UP BY DOZE*. I cad feel it ride *heeerrre*," as she pointed emphatically to her left sinus with an anxious flourish. The translation, read with utter disdain, is as follows: "No, *MOM*, I got a flip-flop up my *NOSE*. A Polly Pocket flip-flop *UP MY NOSE*. I can feel it right *heeerrre*." And then it made sense why our off-season clothes weren't the issue here.

For those of you unschooled in the world of Polly Pocket (which thankfully I, too, had been until just prior to the incident at hand), they are these teeny little Barbie Dolls that would easily fit—I know this is a stretch, here—into even the most miniscule of pockets. Thus, the name Polly Pocket. Aside from their size, though, the unique thing about these dolls is that they come with no less than 750,000 wee accessories like purses, bracelets, brushes, mini (and I *do* mean mini) skirts, and yes, you guessed it, tiny blue flip-flops. I'm convinced that these dolls were invented by a collaborative of vacuum cleaner manufacturers and toy companies for the dual purpose of testing the hardiness of new vacuum models (since the only places those accessories are effectively stored is at the bottom of a hurricane-action canister vac), and ensuring that the doll manufacturer has a built-in sales strategy to perpetually fill replacement orders. Through her fear and pain (I mean, it's gotta hurt, right?), Malina was weeping uncontrollably and begging us to help her get it out.

All the while, I can only imagine how this whole thing

transpired . . . Malina sitting on the family room floor, bored and ready for action, when she stumbles across this tiny blue flip-flop. She picks it up, examines it, and nonchalantly says, "Huh . . . it's a tiny blue flip-flop." After rotating it a couple of times with her nimble kindergarten fingers, she casually considers, "Hmmm . . . I wonder where that might fit," glancing slightly up to the side imagining the infinite possibilities (which, I'm sure, included no fewer options than the DVD player, an electrical socket, one of my lipstick tubes, the kitchen faucet, and her father's nose-hair trimmer). Lips slightly pursed, she settled on the most convenient of her options: right in the middle of her face. "I wonder if it might fit up my nose." After another dramatic pause, with an uncommon blend of inquisitiveness and nonchalance, she makes her decision. "Maybe I'll try it," and proceeds to gingerly insert said flip-flop into her nasal cavity. With certainty and conviction she congratulates herself, "Yep, just like I thought. It *does* fit. I was right." Pleased by her remarkably accurate call, she continues, "Well, that was fun. I think I'll go ahead and take it out now." And the "uh oh" portion of our program begins.

I imagine that she was concerned about our potential response to this situation, since we had (like all parents), cautioned her for years against inserting foreign objects of any kind into receptacles that were not expressly made for their storage. As such, it appears that she may have spent quite some time trying to get that thing out of there, because by the time she got to us, the wayward piece of footwear was nowhere to be found. I took over soggy baby detail and turned the sleuthing over to Dad. "Michael, you're going to have to see if you can find it, because I think that thing's wedged up there in her skull somewhere." Michael sighed heavily, his stress and irritation escalating by the minute.

Now, Michael and I deal with stress very differently, which typically yields a whole yin/yang balance thing that results in better outcomes in *most* situations. This was decidedly *not* one of those instances. He looked at me with great exasperation and cried, "*Why* would she *do* that?!" I responded with what I thought was an obvious and objective assessment of the situation: "Hmmm, because she's *five*, and she wondered whether it would fit up her *nose* and she's so stinkin' *smart* that she found she was *right* and it *did*." He glared at me and initiated his examination.

What ensued was kind of like watching a really inept Cirque du Soleil performance, with all of the contortions and drama of the real thing but without any grace or identifiable skill. As I've shared with my audiences and readers, the only way to describe Michael is that he's "a really big dude." Sort of football player big. For some unknown reason—call it stress or temporary insanity—instead of having Malina sit or lay down, Michael proceeded to kneel below her and contort his fifty-year-old body like a gymnast (sans flexibility or small stature) to stoop underneath the diminutive nose of a roughly four-foot-tall five-year-old. It was a sight to behold. He's writhing around, trying to get the right angle to peer into her tiny sinus and (go figure) he can't see a darn thing. He says, "Hold on, I'll be right back," and shuffles down the hall. He returns with the smallest flashlight I've ever seen. I couldn't tell if it was part of some sort of Polly Pocket Cat Burglar accessory set or if it was supposed to be a key ring (I imagine the latter), but in either case, it's size was even further dwarfed in his massive hands. He could barely pinch the little button to turn it on, but somehow managed to do so and returned (yes, again) to his bizarre *Crouching Tiger, Hidden Dragon* position underneath Malina. I half expected slow-motion martial arts choreography to ensue.

"I don't see it," he fumed, standing up again. "I don't believe this. You know, if we can't get that thing *out* of there, we're going to have to take her into the *ER* and they're going to have to *take* it out." This statement, as you might imagine, was received rather poorly by Malina, who inherited a sense of drama far beyond her five years. I'm paraphrasing here, but I believe her response was, "Noooooooo . . . Daddy . . . they'rrre gonnnnnnaaaaa haaaaavvvveee to take it ouuuuuttttt?" It was a whine/wail/whinny combination, which was wickedly grating. I'm quite certain she was imagining the ER staff using the Jaws of Life to pry open her nasal cavity to expose the wedged flip-flop, which they would then extract using nothing less than a backhoe. She was shaking now, and her voice had effectively approximated the screech of a flock of seagulls in that cramped bathroom.

As the stress seemed to be getting to everyone, we decided that a change of venue might be in order, so we all slogged back into the family room to continue with the excavation mission. Michael downshifted to low-tones mode in an effort to calm Malina down. "Okay, Malina," he whispered reassuringly, "I'm sure we'll be able to take care of this, no problem. Just relax." He sounded like a cross between an NPR radio announcer and a slasher movie psycho-killer just before he cracks. It was eerie, but she seemed to respond well and, after a few mutual deep breaths, they both calmed down enough for him to proceed.

(Note to self: Utilize NPR/psycho-killer voiceover when prepping Malina for annual flu shot.)

I felt like I'd held it together pretty well through the ordeal, but the ratio of absurdity to normalcy had finally tipped the scale. And so, as they engaged in team yogic breathing, at what may have been one of the *least* opportune moments (though were there really any *more* opportune moments?), I *laughed*. And laughed. And laughed some more. Michael, still squatting on the floor in a quasi-artistic rendering of a piece titled, "The Great Indignity," looked up at me with a degree of disdain reserved only for the most heinous of marital spats. "*Why* are you *laughing*?" he spit out between clenched teeth. Ah, the familiar taste of venom. Since it always seems to taste better with salt, I responded by rubbing a little into the wound and shared the only comment I felt was called for in the moment. "Why *aren't* you *laughing*?"

Malina glanced at me, shocked and stunned. I could see her mentally tabulating the therapy bills that one day she would package up and send to me with a note that simply reads, "*You* started this. *You* pay for it." She would then pen a scathing letter about how all of her dysfunction, including the loss of her sense of smell during stressful interludes, can be traced back to "the blue flip-flop incident," from which she would have readily recovered had I not uncontrollably laughed during the critical moment rather than offering reassurance, compassion, and unconditional love. (In my defense, those things were all there. They were just impossible to discern through my rather obnoxious display of hysteria.)

Michael returned to the task at hand with renewed conviction, which seemed to pay off because almost immediately he sounded the triumphant battle cry, "I think I see it! I see something *blue*! Deenie, get me the tweezers!" which he followed with a flourished wave of his arm. Once again, Malina, who at this point in her life did not even know what tweezers *were* (yet surmised that they must involve great pain and unbearable discomfort), donned her most dramatic of voices to moan, "Nooooooo, daddddddyyyyyy . . . not the tweeeezzzzeeeerrrrrssss . . ." after which she proceeded to collapse into a heap on the floor, sobbing and shaking.

Michael kept himself in check and said, "Okay, Malina, we'll try this *one more time*. I'm going to cover *this* side of your nose and count to three. When I get to three, I want you to blow as hard as you can through the *other* side of your nose, okay?" "Okay, Daddy, just pppplllllleeeeeaaaasssseeee don't use the twwwweeeezzzzeerrrrs." Highly motivated by now, she braced herself for the mother of all nose blows. "Okay, Mal," Michael cooed, again in the NPR/psycho-killer voice. "Here we go. One . . . two . . . THREE," at which time she let out a honk like a war siren, making me want to take cover under the kitchen table. It was a truly stunning sinus-purging extravaganza.

In fact, she was *so* motivated (another note to self: threaten the use of tweezers for other incidents requiring behavior modification) that that blue flip-flop came flying out of there at *ninety miles an hour*. I'm serious. You could have stopped a speeding freight train with the force of that blue Polly Pocket flip-flop. The recoil was enough to cause her to lose her balance before haphazardly rebounding to her starting position. She raised her eyebrows in both surprise and relief, and sighed, "It's *out*!" I half expected to see a miniature Polly Pocket marching band leading a festive ticker-tape parade through the room after the whole ordeal.

At about that time, my nephew, Jacob, who had been obliviously sitting on the floor watching some television show throughout the whole event, leapt up from his seat, ran over to assess the carnage, eyes wide with anticipation. "Can *I* see it?" After examining the wreckage he nonchalantly offered, "I've seen worse," and returned to his seat without another word. Flip-flop extraction completed. Child removed from harm's way. Husband in need of chiropractic adjustment. Marriage possibly in jeopardy. Future of the psychotherapy profession ensured (since Malina will no doubt become a lifelong client of some lucky counselor as a result of this incident). My work here is done.

A SLICE OF INSIGHT:
BLOW OUT THOSE FLIP-FLOPS

Malina recovered (at least physically) from the incident almost immediately and vowed to keep all foreign objects a safe distance from her sinuses. But the whole ordeal got me thinking, "How many of us are carrying around blue flip-flops in uncomfortable places in our lives?" How many of us have looked at something and, for whatever reason, thought to ourselves, "Yeah . . . *I think I can make that fit*." It could be an unwanted commitment, an old way of thinking, something we added to our schedule, another committee, an unproductive habit, or a toxic relationship. Basically, those blue flip-flops are defined as anything that doesn't serve our best interests and the best interests of all involved.

You can often identify blue flip-flops by the sheer discomfort they create in your life, usually by way of frustration, exhaustion, or resentment (or all three). For instance, if you're the team member who stays late at the office to finish the projects 90 percent of the time, if you're the neighbor who hosts all the kids at your house 90 percent of the time, or if you're the life partner who takes care of 90 percent of the household duties, it's no wonder you may start to feel (and respond to) the distress caused by that imbalance. Blue flip-flops can be one-sided friendships or two-faced colleagues, too many meetings or too much "stuff," worrying about others' opinions or worrying about what you cannot change. It's healthy to identify those things that *don't* bring value or joy into your life so you can thoughtfully replace them with things that *do*. You can create an amazing amount of space in your schedule, home, work, relationships, and (best of all) your *mind* when you release what *doesn't* serve you and redirect your focus and resources to something that *does*.

> **Y**ou can create an amazing amount of space in your schedule, home, work, relationships, and (best of all) your *mind* when you release what *doesn't* serve you and redirect your focus and resources to something that *does*.

That's when, just like Malina, we can come to the realization that, "Just because I was originally able to fit something *into* my life, doesn't necessarily mean that I have to *keep* it there." That can be the tough part. Malina learned that it can be a lot easier to wedge something into a tight spot than it is to get it back out again. The same often holds true for us. It tends to be a lot easier to *acquire* an ill-placed blue flip-flop in our lives than it can be to identify how it's not serving us anymore and then figure out how to let it go.

Blue flip-flop extraction requires two very important steps. First, it requires that you pay attention to the things in your life that are filling your *mind* with satisfying thoughts, your *schedule*

> The average outcome from the way we spend our time, energy, and ultimately our life, should yield more fulfillment than frustration.

with meaningful activities, and your *soul* with purposeful joy. That doesn't mean that we necessarily like *every* minute of *every* day or *every* task of *every* commitment, but it does mean that the average outcome from the way we spend our time, energy, and ultimately our life, should yield more fulfillment than frustration. Once you've stepped up your awareness about what should *stay* (those things that enrich your life) and what should *go* (those things that deplete your reserves), you've got to take *action*. That's when, rather than resorting either to drama or to victimhood, it's time to take swift and productive steps to change what you can. Respectfully resign from

> Once you've stepped up your awareness about what should *stay* (those things that enrich your life) and what should *go* (those things that deplete your reserves), you've got to take *action*.

the committee. Politely decline the next get-together with that toxic friend. Schedule the next playdate at the neighbors' home instead of yours. Specifically request your family's help with the household tasks. When you find a blue flip-flop and decide it's time to release it, you, too, can blow that baby out of there at ninety miles an hour. Brace yourself, take a deep breath, and blow!

MINDFULNESS BITE BY BITE: FLIP-FLOP PROPULSION PRACTICES

1. What "blue flip-flops" are you carting around in your life? (Remember, these could be old ways of thinking, commitments, people, habits, schedule conflicts, or other things that don't serve your best interests and the best interests of all involved.)

2. Select one of those flip-flops and identify how you will *feel* (relieved, peaceful, free, energized) when you have effectively released it from your life. (Be as detailed as you can!)

3. With that same flip-flop in mind, list the number of ways you will *benefit* from blowing it out of your life. How will you redirect that time, energy, and emotion in ways that will enhance your life and bring more joy to both you and others?

Backup Panties

After I started analyzing my own life for stray blue flip-flops, I identified a number of things that I could benefit from "releasing" (diplomatic term) or "blowing out of my life at ninety miles per hour" (more accurate term). I kept asking myself, "What do I want to let go of that isn't serving me? What clouds my thinking, my energy, my sense of peace, and my happiness?

Which flip-flop does not belong?" While I identified a number of things that needed to be blown out of my life—old ways of thinking, commitments that brought more stress than joy, relationships that had become unfulfilling—I decided that there were too many to take on at once. Since I didn't want to stress myself out in my attempt to de-stress (amen to that!), I simply asked myself, "What *one* thing could I let go of that would make an immediate, tremendous positive difference in my life?" It came to me like a flash of genius, flooding me with an immediate sense of calm repose. And then it buried me in a heap of unwashed clothing. I blew out my laundry.

I regularly confide in my audiences my alternating distaste for and disinterest in housekeeping of all kinds. In fact, it's probably one of the things that elicits the most rowdy chorus of "amens" when I share it with the audiences who attend my comedy show. I actually have to discipline myself to host an occasional family event or in-home gathering because that's the only thing that rallies me to bring the house into any sense of order, and it has the extra benefit of helping me maintain a basic adherence to the local public health ordinances.

I take pride in the fact that, at least as this book goes to print, I have not yet been reported to Child Protective Services for not only allowing my kids to exercise the "five-second rule" in my home but for extending it into time periods that may eventually result in their inexplicable diagnosis of mad cow disease, their unfortunate development of gangrene in one or more limbs, or their suffering through inexplicable bone loss of nefarious origin. I'm quite certain that with this admission, I will no longer be trusted by the parents of my children's friends to host playdates or slumber parties. Another blue flip-flop effectively blown clear of my perimeter.

It's true that I will never win a *Good Housekeeping* award (or "Moderately Acceptable Housekeeping," or even "Bordering on Passable Housekeeping," for that matter). This is because, when faced with the choice of loading the dishwasher, dust-mopping the floor, or folding the laundry, I will undoubtedly choose other activities infinitely more *soul-filling*, like snuggling my children, enjoying a glass of wine and deep conversation with my husband, or learning something meaningful and life-changing. In all honesty, I'd also be more likely to forgo housekeeping in favor of other activities infinitely more pleasure-seeking in the moment, like *eating ice cream* with my children, enjoying a glass of wine and *superficial* conversation with my husband, or learning something *completely useless and just plain fun*, like how to spell inappropriate words upside down on a calculator.

True, chores are fairly low on my list of things I willingly do, falling roughly between watching almost any reality TV program and submitting myself for a frontal lobotomy. I finally realized that doing the laundry wasn't creating any meaning, purpose, or joy for me, and everyone else noticed, too. In fact, just recently Michael and I were talking about the things that we appreciate about one another, and the last thing he mentioned (after providing me with an inventory of the many things that make me so darned fabulous . . . was it wrong to ask him to annotate and sign the list?) was the following: "I really appreciate that you do the laundry. Wait. I mean, I really appreciate that you *attempt* to do the laundry." What a eulogy that would be. "Deanna Davis. Loving wife, mother, sister, friend. Accomplished author, speaker, and entertainer. Lover of chocolate, cheese, and cabernet. And she attempted to do the laundry." Just gives you the warm fuzzies all over, doesn't it?

But after the ego blow, I got the message: Not only was laundry an energy drain and an irritation for me, I obviously wasn't very *good* at it, either. So I decided to renounce trying to act like I actually *cared* about that dreaded task. Instead, I directed my focus toward something that could yield a more positive benefit for me (like taking a nap) or could at least be more entertaining (like learning how to train picnic ants to do Super Bowl–type halftime shows).

So, here's where it stands now: I don't make any real attempt at all to keep up with the laundry. I sort of let it pile up until no one in the house has anything left to wear. Wait, let me clarify. Until *I* don't have anything left to wear, or, more specifically, until I've nearly made my way through my stash of "backup panties." People look at me with great disdain when I bring up backup panties. But let's be honest, everyone has them.

Backup panties are the ones you wear when all the others are gone. The ones that you've had since junior high (which incidentally cut off most of the critical circulation both to your reproductive organs and to your lower extremities), or are either (1) so big that you could show a drive-in movie on them, or (2) so stretched out that they resemble a white flag of surrender rather than undergarments. They're your last-ditch dainties, the ones that you pray you won't be wearing in the event you ever get into an accident because if the trauma didn't kill you, the humiliation of the emergency medical team seeing you in your backup panties most assuredly would. Yes, we all have them. In fact, many of us are probably wearing them this very moment. You know who you are (and now you all know who I am, too). So, anyway, once I'm to the last pair of backup panties it's time to immerse myself in a full-day "power wash." It's kind of like tax season, only it sadly comes around a lot more frequently than once a year (most of the time, at least).

Even though I've instituted the power wash cycle, it appears that I may still have some kind of psychological block against actually putting away the resulting mounds of textiles. Piles of laundry, sometimes folded, often not, find their way to an assortment of locations throughout the house, but they rarely wind up in the right place or with the right person. This became crystal clear one day when Malina, age six at the time, bounded up to me and innocently asked, "Mommy, have you seen my pink pants? I looked in the stack in my room, the load in the dryer, the pile on the dining room table, that batch on the living room couch, the basket on your closet floor, and the stuff on your bathroom counter and I can't find them *anywhere*." "Well," I said with one of those "Hello? Aren't you missing something?" kind of tones in my voice, "Did you think to try looking in your *dresser drawers*?" With only the slightest pause and a rather impatient tone, she replied, "Well, why on *earth* would they be in *there*?"

I'd like to say I was shocked by her response, but I wasn't. I knew this day would come. I reasoned that I had actually done her a service by enacting my laundry boycott, because it taught her tenacity, self-sufficiency, and the rigorous application of deductive reasoning to succeed in life. Yes, this girl will be a survivor. Perhaps a survivor attired entirely in dry-clean-only apparel, but a survivor nonetheless.

My son, on the other hand, may not fare so well in our "clean laundry deprivation chamber." Though his sister was dubbed the "mission impossible baby," exceptionally motivated, hardy, and willing to do whatever she needed to do to master *anything* simply for the thrill of the challenge, my son was dubbed "Reggae boy," because he primarily just wants to "hang with his peeps" and listen to music. Case in point: The boy didn't roll over until he was nine months old, an issue I finally felt merited a quick question to Carsten's nurse practitioner. She assessed him and objectively reported: "He's strong, healthy, and developing just fine. He's just . . . well . . . chubby. It takes a lot of momentum to move that much mass." I beg to differ. I think it was because he knew that once he *did* roll over he'd have to expend the energy to keep doing it for his entire life so he figured he'd hold out until it was absolutely necessary, say, until it became critical to secure his next meal.

That being said, I can't imagine him seeking out clean clothes from seventeen unique locations in our home, and thus can imagine him simply walking around in togas made of dishrags, or cleverly concealing his most delicate regions with a series of strategically placed Matchbox cars rather than inconveniencing himself to seek out an appropriate (and hygienic) outfit. But I have some time to solve that one. Maybe by then I'll have figured out how to release my concern about what other people think about my *parenting skills* and just applaud his creativity and self-sufficiency when he's able to clothe himself entirely in his sister's unused hair scrunchies. Prepare for another blue flip-flop launch!

A SLICE OF INSIGHT:
LETTING GO OF THE LAUNDRY

I have to say that the blowing-out of my laundry flip-flop was liberating. I no longer needed to make excuses about *when* I would do it or *why* it wasn't done or *where* anything was. And, I no longer needed to pretend that it was even the slightest bit important to me. Instead, that extra energy went toward things I care more about, like enjoying meals with my family and reading just a little more often, playing with the kids, or helping others in need. Okay, it's true that *some* of the energy went toward just trying to find my clothes after power wash Wednesday, but I'm willing to compromise a bit of efficiency here and there to experience more of what I want in life! It seems that each time we release a begrudging "should" from our lives it makes space for an emphatic "good!" of some kind . . . something to honor, celebrate, or cherish (or all three). That release not only *feels* a lot better, but it also *achieves* a lot more for the people we care about in our lives.

> Each time we release a begrudging "should" from our lives it makes space for an emphatic "good!" of some kind . . . something to honor, celebrate, or cherish (or all three). That release not only *feels* a lot better, but it also *achieves* a lot more for the people we care about in our lives.

This whole idea of deciding what to let go of has to do with "opportunity costs" and "tradeoffs." In this case, opportunity costs are the things that you could have done instead of what you decided to do—the things that you gave up in order to do something else. They are the things that you could have chosen to spend your precious resources (like time, energy, and focus) on, if you wanted to. Tradeoffs are what you are willing to compromise on in order to choose one option over another. These are the things that might be *nice* but not *necessary* to you at this point in time, or the things that you may *value*—sometimes dearly—but you simply don't value them *as much* as an alterna- tive. Value is the key, and you get to decide what you value more in a given moment. Knowing you have a choice is the ultimate in self-direction.

> **V**alue is the key, and you get to decide what you value more in a given moment. Knowing you have a choice is the ultimate in self-direction.

So, for some people, getting the laundry done brings them significant value, perhaps in terms of *feelings* (maybe they feel organized, that they are providing a meaningful service or a good environment for their family, or like they have achieved something). Or, it may bring them value in terms of *schedule* and *space* resources (maybe they like being able to easily and efficiently find what they need). Or possibly, they value the im- pact of their laundry outcomes on either *stress levels* or *rela- tionships*. (Maybe it decreases stress in the household to have things orderly, and maybe family members feel cared for when this task is taken care of.) More power to them (and more power wash to them, as well!). That's the cool thing—each per- son, each family, and each organization gets to make their own decisions about what they value most. Then they get to create their experiences according to those values. And those decisions will vary just like our body types and personality styles—they are all unique. Some people might look at the idea of opportunity costs and tradeoffs as something negative—like they lost out on something in the course of choosing something else—but I suggest that there's a more empowering interpretation of these concepts. Opportunity costs and tradeoffs provide you with the ultimate in decision-making power because they provide *contrast* that helps you choose a course of action based on what's *important* to you . . . they are all about living by *design* rather than by *default*.

> Opportunity costs and tradeoffs provide you with the ultimate in decision-making power because they provide *contrast* that helps you choose a course of action based on what's *important* to you . . . they are all about living by *design* rather than by *default*.

In my household, we do our best to consciously move from default to design when we can. Sure, we need to have clean clothes at some point, but we don't need to have them in the way that society, or my far more laundry-capable neighbors, or those perky laundry detergent commercials dictate. We can have them in *our own* way in *our own* sweet time. (Or maybe in *my own* way in *my own* sweet time?) In the meantime, we'll have our meals together . . . and our playtime . . . and our homework sessions . . . and our wine and conversations . . . and every few weeks we'll have a power wash day together, too. Seems to work for us. What will you find works for you?

We all have our blue flip-flops and backup panties. From one-sided friendships to two-faced colleagues, from too many meetings to too much "stuff" in your space,

> Life will provide you with ample opportunities to *release* what doesn't serve you and *redirect* your focus and resources to something that *does*.

and from worrying about others' opinions to worrying about what you can't change, life will provide you with ample opportunities to *release* what doesn't serve you and *redirect* your focus and resources to something that *does*. When you don't exactly know what to *do* but you know things aren't as you'd like them to *be*, it might be time to blow out one of those flip-flops and embrace your inner backup panties. Rest assured, your wardrobe choices might suffer but you certainly won't be sorry.

MINDFULNESS BITE BY BITE: CATCH AND RELEASE

1. Where in your life are you holding on to doing something, being something, or acting in some way that causes you significant *opportunity costs*?

2. What *tradeoffs* are you willing to make to let go of those things that are causing you so many opportunity costs in order to experience something better?

3. In the future, what checks and balances can you set up to *catch* yourself in the act of doing something you'd be better off not doing, and how will you commit to *release* it from your life?

Wandering Weasels

We had just moved into our new home, which I refer to as our "little house on the prairie," primarily because, well, it sits on a prairie. I've never lived in a rural area before, so I'm finding that there are all sorts of adventures you can have just going about your business while ten acres of land plot against you, waiting for the moment that you turn your back so you can learn things, like the fact that when there are power outages wells simply don't work (and you also discover the huge volumes of water you feel you need for one reason or another when you don't have access to it).

Or, there are revelations that appear in the form of massive snowdrifts, through which you learn that when it snows several feet over the course of a couple of days, a family can easily wedge its small SUV into a snow pile of colossal proportions in their own driveway, tiny children in tow, with nothing to feed them but stale holiday candy. You discover that you can continue providing such a diet until a gracious friend makes his way through the blizzard to help dig your misplaced metro family out of the snowdrift since the entire county is in a state of emergency and no one who gets paid to help you will actually come to do so. (Incidentally, I've found that small children find interludes like these infinitely satisfying, but be forewarned that infusing tiny bodies with nothing but refined sugar and subsequently containing them in a very small space for long periods of time is ill advised. For the record, it is indeed possible for a one-year-old boy to serve as music conductor to a car full of people singing "John Jacob Jinglehimer Schmidt" ad nauseum, which alone would be only barely tolerable, but fueled by an all-sugar diet, it becomes a form of inhumane torture, with your only respite being the sounds of him squealing like a starving, agitated piglet at any attempt to influence the playlist.

And then there's the whole critter issue. On the day in question, I was sitting in the office of my new home, madly writing and editing in order to meet the publishing deadline for my previous book (*The Law of Attraction in Action*), which just happened to be due the week before an even more important due date—the birth of my baby boy, Carsten. A bit loopy from sustaining myself on a diet of word soup and pregnancy hormones for too long, I sensed I wasn't alone in the room, and hoped that maybe my husband had ventured in to deliver a cup of tea or a shoulder rub. I looked up a bit distractedly from the computer to spy not a doting husband but a prairie critter of some kind standing on his hind legs in the doorway, casually gazing at me. He wasn't startled or scared. He wasn't even really intrigued (which I found disturbing in itself, as I find myself particularly fascinating). He just looked at me with this nonchalant expression that seemed to say, "Hey . . . lady. What's up?"

I shifted in my seat as I surveyed the situation. Now, I'm a product of suburbia, where the most common furry guests I would find on our property were well-groomed, entitlement-oriented Generation X house pets skulking around to see if the grass really was greener on the other side of the fence (which I assure you that in *our* case was categorically false). As such, I know nothing about critters of any kind, and though for a wild creature, this one looked like he had a rather pleasant demeanor, I've heard through the prairie grass-vine that some of them can be quite vicious. I didn't want to take any chances. And, I really needed to get back to my writing. Since I couldn't see where the little beast would have had occasion to acquire any editorial expertise or copyediting skills on the range, I didn't feel the need to welcome him in.

For a brief moment I explored my options. I decided that a

calm, rational conversation might yield the best results, so in my most pleasant voice, I said, "Hello, little critter. You don't belong in here. Will you please leave now?" He looked at me as if to say, "I don't mean to be rude, but I'm not sure if you realize how ridiculous you look making small talk with vermin," and then promptly turned around and headed into the laundry room, which seemed fitting based on my previous admissions about the state of the laundry. I got up and followed him in there, where he stood between the door to the garage and the washing machine, an apathetic expression on his face. I tried again. "Would you please leave, now, because we only have enough bedrooms for our family members, so I really don't have space for you. Thanks for stopping by." He tilted his head as if to say, "Lady . . . what don't you *get*? I am a wild animal, tiny but filthy and feisty. Do I look civilized to you? Are you planning on giving me a grammar lesson next?"

I sensed his confusion (or was it annoyance?) so I resorted to sign language. I pointed to the door with a warm and gentle flourish to make it look really appealing, kind of like a game show host suggesting, "And behind door number three . . . *your freedom*!" "Why don't you just go out that door." I smiled. "It's really easy . . . I do it every day. And you can, too. All you have to do is make the choice. It's all about choice." And now I realize that, through that last comment, I may have just hatched a concept for a new reality-television series called *The Choice: True Tales of Varmint Intervention*. I could have sworn I saw him roll his eyes and shake his teeny, bristly head. So, I called in the reinforcements.

I shouted to our builder, who was in the garage doing something builder-esque. "Allen," I said, "there's a critter in the house. Can you help me get him out?" He ambled around the corner. "Oh yeah . . . him. He's a little weasel. Isn't he cute?" "Well, yes, Allen, he is indeed cute," I responded. Allen continued, "And he eats the mice, too, which is a good thing." "That's great, Allen," I responded, "that he's both cute *and* functional. What a wonderful combination. But I still don't want him taking up residence in my house. I've carefully chosen the family members I'd like to live with, and they don't include varmints of any kind. In fact, my husband barely made the cut. I want him gone. Can you help?" "Got it," he said, and he gently helped shoo the wandering weasel out of the laundry room and back to his home on the range.

A SLICE OF INSIGHT: SEIZING WEASELS

As I reflected on the incident later on, I thought about Allen's observation that the little weasel was most certainly cute, and that, in his role as an unassuming mouse-terminator, he was also most assuredly functional. And yet, he didn't belong in my home. He belonged prowling the prairie, not lounging in my unwashed laundry. I got to thinking about how many other wandering weasels we tend to allow into our lives—habits and ways of think-

> It pays to be mindful about whether or not our existing habits of thinking and acting are yielding substantial benefit in our lives. If they aren't, it's time to change them. Habits are incredibly valuable provided they are healthy and helpful . . . not a hindrance.

ing that might be cute and/or functional (or both)—that belonged in our *past* or in other *circumstances* or in other areas of our *lives*, but that don't belong where they are *right now*.

Let's consider habits for a moment. The role of a *constructive* habit is to put certain behaviors on autopilot in order to save focus and energy for the things that most deserve our *conscious attention*. It pays to be mindful about whether or not our existing habits of thinking and acting are yielding substantial benefit in our lives. If they aren't, it's time to change them. Habits are incredibly valuable provided they are healthy and helpful . . . not a hindrance.

What habits do *you* have that might be functional elsewhere but don't necessarily belong in a certain area of your life? For example, what about your time? Do you keep a relatively structured schedule to make sure that your kids get to their school and extracurricular activities, but does that rigidity keep you from carving out time for yourself? Do you have a phenomenal work ethic that produces outstanding results on the job, but which at times prevents you from taking much-deserved breaks to recharge? Have you developed habits with your focus, time, or energy that served you in a previous phase of your life (in college, before you were a homeowner, or when you had more free time) but that actually infringe on your quality of life now because they keep you from being in the moment or experiencing what you want to?

What about your ways of *thinking*? Are there aspects of your mind-set that serve you in certain circumstances, but not others? For instance, are you successful in your profession because you can be objective and analytical, but does that create strife in your marriage because it keeps you from connecting on an emotional level? Are you known for your self-deprecating sense of humor with all of your friends, but does that translate to being overly harsh and judgmental of yourself? Are you very relaxed and "go with the flow" in your personal life, which feels great, but does that same mentality cause perpetual money struggles for you because you have no structure for your financial well-being?

These are just a few examples of the "wandering weasels" that can make their way into our minds—and our lives—unbidden. I'm sure you can identify a slew of others that exist in your life (and I assure you I can, too). Sometimes, it's simply the *awareness* of such a weasel that can help you decide what you want to do with it. At times, maybe a rational conversation with yourself will work (even though it didn't work for my weasel, it's certainly worth a try!). Other times, just the act of pulling your game-show flourish to escort it out of your experience will do. And, with others, you may need to call in the reinforcements to help you usher the weasel to more appropriate venues. In any case, this process of releasing starts with identifying something that *doesn't* belong in your life and ushering it *out* so you can feel comfortable and content again. So, why not focus on stewarding your wandering weasels to their appropriate environments and consciously choose who—and *what*—you want to invite in to your life?

> This process of releasing starts with identifying something that *doesn't* belong in your life and ushering it *out* so you can feel comfortable and content again.

MINDFULNESS BITE BY BITE:
USHERING OUT WHAT DOESN'T BELONG

1. What habitual ways of thinking, acting, or being just aren't serving your best interests anymore?

2. What is your plan and support system to help usher those unproductive things out of your life?

3. What new habitual way of thinking or acting will you establish to create better results for yourself in the future?

CHAPTER 7

Mindfulness and the "Moment-ous" Life

Apple of My Pie

It's fitting to introduce this *last* chapter talking about the *first* thing that introduced me to the concept of mindfulness: apple pie. As I described in Chapter 1, the *process* of making that very first pie and the *product* of its impact on my life (a significant number of extra pounds notwithstanding) directly led to my commitment to living a "moment-ous" life. A "moment-ous" life is just that—a series of moments, one after the other, when we *purposely choose to be in the here and now*. This is no small task, when there are so many opportunities to live in the past, regretting what we did or didn't do, or to live in the future, presuming that it will somehow be better or easier or more appealing than the present. It takes conviction to be mindful. And it takes patience. And practice.

To be fully here is to let go of the flawed assumption that any other place, time, or situation is more "right" for you than this one. It doesn't matter whether your "now" is filled with energy and eagerness, peace and prosperity, or hardship and heartache, it only matters that you are *present in it* to learn what you're meant to learn and to experience what you're meant to experience. But if you're like me, I imagine you'd strongly prefer to feel *positive* rather than *negative* emotions, and to experience *pleasant* things rather than *unpleasant* ones. This always reminds me of a quote from a very wise person, who once said, "Well, *duh!*" Of *course* the good stuff always *feels* better to us and we want to have more, more, more of it, please. Who wouldn't? But that's just not the reality of life. In polite terms, "stuff happens," and it's a good thing it does sometimes because (as I discussed in *The Law of Attraction in Action*), we need *contrast* in our lives to help us *delight* in what we have, *define* what we want to experience more of, and *decide* what we want to change. Unless you have comparisons, you'd live your life never knowing *what* to change, *why* you want to change it, or *how* the heck to go about changing it.

As such, the following stories explore the concepts of mindfulness and contrast to help you create your *own* definition of what it means to live a "moment-ous" life. Before we get in to that (of course), we'll take this opportunity to celebrate the power of pastry one last time, and we'll do that with the apple of my pie. I mean, with my apple pie. That's where it all started, and we could say that's where it all ends, but in fact (as you well know by now), this is where it all *begins*.

Apple Pie

1 cup refined sugar

1 cup brown sugar

1 teaspoon cinnamon

½ teaspoon salt

3 tablespoons flour

Pastry for a double-crust pie

9–10 apples (I prefer Granny Smith or a combination of Granny Smith and McIntosh)

¼ cup (½ stick) unsalted butter, cut into small pieces

Ice cream, whipped cream, or sharp Cheddar cheese, optional

Line oven with foil or "drip catcher," or have a baking sheet handy to catch drips from the baking pie. Preheat oven to 475 degrees.

In a mixing bowl, combine sugars, cinnamon, salt, and flour. Mix well and set aside.

Line a pie plate with a pie crust. Peel and core the apples and cut them into thin slices. (As you know, I have a long-standing love affair with my Pampered Chef apple peeler/corer/slicer, so this is what I use and this is what I suggest that everyone use because it will not only bring you great joy but also easy pie preparation. But you can do it the hard way, too. Whatever works for you!)

Place a layer of apples in the bottom of the pie plate. Sprinkle with sugar mixture and dot with butter (equivalent of 1 tablespoon). Continue with at least 4 layers of apples, sugar mixture, and butter. Top with remaining pie crust, seal, and flute the edges. Cut slits to vent.

Cover edges of crust with foil. Bake for 20 minutes. Remove foil, reduce heat to 400 degrees, and bake for another 20 minutes. Reduce heat again to 350 degrees for 20 minutes or until crust is golden brown and apples are cooked through.

Serve with ice cream, whipped cream, or warm with sharp Cheddar cheese (especially good for breakfast!) and as you take the first bite, celebrate this moment and your commitment to living a mindful, "moment-ous" life!

Misdirected Multitasking

I'm rather well known in my circle for my utter incapacity to do two things at once. The whole "can't walk and chew gum" thing applies here. While I pride myself in knowing and capitalizing on my strengths (like the ability to direct rapt focus on what's in front of me, in which produces great outcomes most of the time), I also acknowledge my unique limitations (such as my complete inability to notice, or attend to, anything other than that one thing, including structures or persons that have become engulfed in flames in my presence). It can actually create disorientation during mundane activities like playing board games.

Case in point: a Trivial Pursuit grudge match between family teams dubbed "The Purveyors of Useless Knowledge" and "The Valedictorians of Minutiae University." My team blatantly ignored my prompt (and, might I add, *correct*) answer to the following question: "What scientific experiment successfully mapped the genetic blueprint of human beings?" They proceeded into an obstacle course of intellectual banter, but I couldn't focus on disputing them because I already knew the answer. It was the Human Genome Project. Just *how* I knew this still remains a mystery to me, but I *did* know that if I lost my train of thought, it would be gone forever and so would, in all likelihood, our chances of winning. So, what transpired sounded something like this:

SISTER: Oh, I know this one.

ME: Human Genome Project.

SON-IN-LAW: It's right on the tip of my tongue.

ME: Human Genome Project.

DAUGHTER: I remember learning about this one in science class.

ME: Human Genome Project.

BROTHER-IN-LAW: I'm pretty sure this is that thing that was on the cover of *Time*.

ME: Human Genome Project.

And so on it went until someone from the other team finally exploded with, "Will you guys *please* respond to Rain Man over here? She's getting on our *nerves!*" Though we did win the game that night, due in part to my expert identification of the most famous genetic research study ever, to this day when we're choosing teams for the family reunion volleyball match they still wager on which team gets the privilege of calling Rain Man its own.

My stepdaughters appreciate that my inability to multitask can be an affordable source of entertainment during tough economic times. When they were still living at home, whenever they were bored and didn't have any spending cash, they would innocently propose that we play a game of "spoons," which, they suggested, was "wholesome family fun." For the uninitiated among you, spoons is a card game that requires nothing more than luck and quick reflexes. There are spoons in the middle of the table that add up to one less than the number of players in the game, a la musical chairs. When one player gets the desired hand, he or she grabs a spoon, triggering the rest of the players to scramble to grab one, too. Now, I know what you're probably thinking: "Sounds pretty benign." And in other, less ruthless families, it very well may be. But in my family, the entire game becomes an exercise in determining how many times my loved ones can make me flinch before I develop a permanent and rather unbecoming twitch and/or recurrent seizures.

Now, the average person can simply play the game, attempt to grab the spoon, and be okay with the whole process regardless of whether they actually grasp the flatware. For me, though, the sheer depth of my focus on the cards turns it into an adrenaline-pumping, cortisol-coursing display of unchecked anxiety. Inevitably, by the time it actually registers in my brain that someone has grabbed a spoon and that I would be wise to, as well, all the other players are already sitting back in their chairs, spoons in hand, sometimes even eating ice cream with them, before I ever actually pry my hands away from the cards. And sometimes they conspire to take turns faking me out, with one darting a hand out there and another monitoring my response time like a mad scientist conducting questionable experiments. And these, my good friends, are the children I've sworn my undying love and adoration to. Do you see why, instead of carbo-loading, I "Chocolate Meltdown Pie–load" before these games? At least it dulls the anxiety response in a mixture of chocolate wrapped in sugar wrapped in fat wrapped in a flaky crust.

But it's not just around the family game table where my multitasking misgivings meet with sad outcomes. No, I'm not that fortunate. For instance, when my husband and I go to Las Vegas, we like to play some of the table games together. But despite acing four quarters' worth of college calculus, I have the simple math capacity of a third grader with an abacus when it comes to basic Blackjack strategy. This is usually no problem, because I'm on the lowest-of-low limit tables where not too many real gamblers find themselves. But I still find ways to make a memorable impression, regardless of where I'm playing. On one occasion it was just Michael, myself, and a dealer who had a dry, crackly voice, and an even drier, cracklier sense of humor. We were playing some game that had an add-on bet that day that required determining if you had a particular set of cards in your hand. If you had them, you would leave your bet as it was, and if you didn't, you could pull back part of your bet, which you indicate by gently scratching your cards on the table as if to "scrape back" your bet.

So, I'm sitting there, calculating my cards on my creaky mental abacus, caterpillaring my eyebrows and chewing on my lower lip. I realize that I didn't have the cards I needed, so I decided to "scrape back" the bet. I waited for the dealer to push it in my direction, all the while calculating and strategizing the next level of play. Continuing to gaze at my cards, I realized she still hasn't pushed my bet back. Again, I scraped and again she did nothing. One last time, I scraped, this time a little louder in an attempt to get her to realize it's time to do her job. Still no chips. I finally looked up to find Michael and the dealer just staring at me.

The dealer had won the hand and cleared the bets quite some time ago. Michael, of course, was immediately cognizant of this fact and he and the dealer had been sitting there chatting with one another, wondering how long it would take for me to figure it out. So now, on occasion when my laser-like focus won't allow me to transition quickly enough for Michael's taste, he simply tucks his tongue to the side of his mouth, cocks his head to the side, and scrapes the table until I respond. And just like my kids, this is the man I get to spend all of eternity with. What a jackpot!

But again, since I'm aware of my strengths and their corresponding "opportunities for improvement," I've chosen a career that supports my need to consciously and creatively refocus on my own terms, so it works pretty well for me. (With, of course, the exception of book signings, when the task of autographing while simultaneously chitchatting tends to result in a large pile of books at each event that are unusable because they are lovingly inscribed with a combination of words I intended to *write* and words I intended to *speak*, such as, "For Janice, what a gorgeous blouse," and "To Stephen, yes I flew into town today.")

Prior to the aha moment when I self-diagnosed my MDD (Multitasking Deficiency Disorder), I still believed that with the right type of training and structure, I, too, would be able to multitask with the best of them. Or at least at family events or in Vegas (I wanted to set attainable goals). During the time in question I was home from work caring for Malina, right in the middle of a potty-training marathon. Malina hadn't quite grasped the concept of the potty chair, which we carted around to every room in the house to help her feel comfortable with it (and to have it close at hand when the need arose). Having recently started her "Daddy and Me" classes at the local gymnastics center, she repurposed the little seat into a pedestal, from which she performed various tumbling moves such as forward rolls, after which she would step up on the stool with a triumphant "ta-da!" to accept her imaginary medal.

I thought it was darned cute, and only once or twice worried about what the neighbors or folks in passing cars would think, since she performed these stunts entirely in the nude with all of the windows open. And then I fast-forwarded to the impact on her life should she ever become an Olympic gymnast. I could hear the sports announcers introducing her with the following commentary: "And now, stepping up to the vault is Malina Paige Davis. Now, Davis has a rather unorthodox approach to her vault routine, but it seems to work for her," at which point she would completely disrobe, step up onto an archaic "Potty Me Perfect" chair and prepare to wow the crowd in more ways than one.

I brought myself back from my reverie as she moved into her beam routine. I absent-mindedly dialed the phone to talk with my colleague about some budget negotiations on a new federal grant we had recently been awarded, all the while watching Malina's warm-up. My colleague put me on hold while she grabbed some documents, and during that time Malina was between events so I took the opportunity to reintroduce her to the more traditional uses of the potty chair.

"Malina, it looks like that chair is really fun for doing gymnastics, but it's actually meant for you to go potty in." "No," she politely replied and continued stretching. "You're a big girl now and you get to go potty like the other big girls do." "No," she retorted again and commenced her warm-up for the floor routine. "*Sissy* goes potty on the toilet," I offered. "No," she said. "*Daddy* goes potty on the toilet." "No." "*Mommy* goes potty on the toilet." But the response I heard wasn't the "No" I expected. Instead, it was, "Well, I'm so glad to hear that. I had often wondered, and I'm thrilled you cleared that up for me."

I turned back to the phone, stuttering and stammering apologies to my colleague, who had returned to the line somewhere halfway through my potty-mouth conversation. And then I turned back to Malina, who had finished her routine with a rather unfortunate (and messy) dismount of sorts. And that's when I decided that multitasking and I just weren't made for one another. I could either negotiate million-dollar budgets or coach my priceless baby, but I'd proven I couldn't do both at the same time.

A SLICE OF INSIGHT: PRODUCTIVITY PRIMER

Multitasking is typically one of those train wrecks waiting to happen for most people. While I joke about my personal inability to do it, research actually *proves* that attempting to multitask is one of the single greatest ways to undermine productivity, work quality, and quality of life—it's just that some people fake it better than others. I am clearly not one of those people. Seriously, though, the brain cannot actually *do* two things at once, so when we try to multitask what we're *really* doing is bouncing back and forth rapidly (or in my case, not so rapidly) between two or more competing areas of focus.

Trying to multitask impacts the mind in a similar way that repeatedly jumping back and forth from one spot to another would impact the body. If you did that, you'd readily exhaust your *body* so you wouldn't be able to perform much of anything effectively (and you'd look pretty ridiculous in the process). Multitasking exhausts the *mind* rapidly, so you

> **A**ttempting to multitask is one of the single greatest ways to undermine productivity, work quality, and quality of life.

lose your ability to focus and you markedly decrease creativity, problem-solving, and both the quality and quantity of work. But since you don't look ridiculous (okay, *some* of us actually *do*), there isn't the obvious clue that the process is working *against* you.

According to researchers at the University of Michigan, the *real* problem is that when you multitask, you have to do two things before you can disengage from the task at hand and engage in a new one. First, you have to make the *decision* to switch tasks and then you have to *stop* using the mental "rules" for the tasks you *were* doing and *start* using new "rules" for what you want to do *now*. That might seem and feel easy when you're doing something superficial like opening the mail while talking on the phone but it starts having more negative effects on both you and what you're trying to accomplish when you're trying to do more complex things that require focus (like, say, negotiating federal grant budgets and potty-training a toddler).

Sometimes the results of multitasking can be *obvious, messy, and embarrassing* (like this experience was for me), sometimes they can be *not so obvious, messy, and counterproductive* (like when you lose critical time on a deadline because you keep checking email each time it beckons), and sometimes they can be *obvious, messy, and dangerous* (like accidents that happen when people try to text while driving). The common denominator for all of these scenarios is that *multitasking is unequivocally messy.* And it almost *never* produces the results you're after.

Multitasking decreases health and increases stress levels, diminishes both quality and quantity of work product, negatively impacts relationships and happiness, and threatens things like profitability and (at times) even lives. Yet we're obsessed—literally addicted—to trying to do more than one thing at a time. What a pity that multitasking, one of the very things people do to try to fit *more* into their schedules and *lives,* is actually causing them to experience *less* of what truly makes life worth *living.* Rather than *mindful living,* multitasking tends to foster *mindless doing.*

> Multitasking, one of the very things people do to try to fit *more* into their schedules and *lives,* is actually causing them to experience less of what truly makes life worth *living.* Rather than *mindful living,* multitasking tends to foster *mindless doing.*

The only certainty we have in this life is the moment we are experiencing *right now.* Why not be in that moment both mindfully and masterfully? Sure, it takes skill and discipline to focus on the here and now instead of the *here* and *there* and *past* and *future* and *now.* But many things we care about, whether they're million-dollar grants or priceless (potty-trained or not) toddlers, are well worth the effort. Mindfulness invites us to be in the present moment, despite the many invitations to visit other ones.

MINDFULNESS BITE BY BITE: MINDLESS DOING VS. MINDFUL LIVING

1. In what areas of your life are you prone to multitasking or missing out on the moment?

2. What specific decision could you make today to transition yourself out of your practice of mindless *doing* and into the practice of mindful *living*?

3. What protections can you put in place in the future to ensure that you will thoughtfully decide both what you will *do* and also how you will *feel* while you're doing it?

This Way to Carson City

I love my job. Big-time. As an author and speaker, I get to spend quality time with amazing people discussing powerful concepts in gorgeous locations. I'm not sure I could be any more satisfied if I were the wine steward in an artisan cheese-and-chocolate factory situated on a beach on Maui (though if they're hiring, I'd entertain an interview just to keep my options open). On this particular day, I had just left a truly transformative weekend working and learning with a group of phenomenal women in McCall, Idaho. McCall is a *breathtaking* location that somehow also manages to help you *catch your breath*. It's a stunning landscape that provides the perfect backdrop for self-discovery. (I must now apologize to my friend and former business manager, Leah, who gravely asked me not to tell this story anymore at the risk of exposing McCall's perfection to the world, as she wants to protect its hidden beauty. Leah, I hope you'll forgive me knowing that this book is intended to serve the greater good.)

In any case, I had spent the weekend as the keynote speaker for the ReCreate McCall Retreat, facilitated by a talented team of women. We were treated to thoughtful gifts and even more thoughtful insights, along with morning yoga, afternoon meditations, and evening meals with fellow attendees you'd certainly want to get to know better. It was a meaningful and memorable event. I had shared with the group principles from my books *The Law of Attraction in Action* and *Living with Intention*, and had also focused on the health-enhancing (and life-enhancing!) power of female connections. Much of what I discussed was about mindfulness and savoring the unique flavor of each life experience. I talked about living purposefully and passionately. And I shared the science-proven benefits of practicing gratitude each day (which, if you're wondering, include less depression and anxiety, better health and relationships, and a big fat boost in happiness levels. Talk about a no-cost, no-hassle miracle drug!).

As I drove out of town I was high on oxytocin, that magical little brain chemical that profoundly relaxes you and mops up the stress hormones in your body. Oxytocin, it seems, is conveniently released free of charge into your system simply by treating yourself to the gift of time with other women. (Yet another cheap and healthy prescription from your internal pharmacy.) Since I truly do practice what I preach, I was completely immersed in the moment, brimming with possibilities, full of vitality, and overflowing with gratitude. I was a mobile waterfall of goodwill. I had a long drive ahead of me, so I settled down to bathe in a little gratefulness.

I started to list the things that I appreciated about my experience that weekend, including the pleasure of a new friendship or two, the privilege of doing what I love, and the pampering of a few extra hours of sleep. And I was so thankful to do all of that in such a beautiful place. As I drove, I realized that everything, absolutely *everything*, seemed so bright and fresh and, well, *new*. I reflected on how powerful this process of mindfulness can be, because in this almost ethereal state, *not one thing* looked the same as when I had driven into McCall several days prior. "Wow, this stuff really works. It's like I'm seeing a whole new landscape," I thought to myself.

As I drove along, enjoying my moments of silent lucidity, I noticed a few signs for Carson City, Nevada. I just figured that these signs were similar to ones I see in several other areas of the Northwest, where you're driving somewhere relatively *close* in proximity and you see signs for somewhere markedly *farther away*, but you just know from experience that you're going to make a turn soon and head in the right direction. So, when you're cruising through Montana and you see a sign for Minneapolis, you know darned well you're going to stop in Billings, exactly 839 miles before the Twin Cities emerge on the horizon. That's what I was *certain* was happening here. I knew I'd get to the turnoff sooner or later and I just wanted to be present in this miraculous moment right here, right now, with nothing else interrupting it.

But the signs to Carson City came more and more frequently, and Nevada loomed closer and closer, with no reference at all to Spokane, Washington. "That's weird," I thought. "McCall, Idaho, is down here"—I pushed a tack into the lower, right side of my mental map—"and Spokane, Washington, is up here"—I pushed a tack into the upper right side on my mental map—"and Carson City is wayyyyyyy over here and wayyyyyy down there"—I pushed a tack into the left, lower corner of my mental map. Just then, another sign indicated that I would arrive in Carson City in relatively short order. In too short order, in fact. And still no reference to Spokane. I pulled over at the next little town and learned a little something about the potential drawbacks to living *too* fully in the present moment.

What I found from the pleasant young man behind the counter was that I had traveled ninety miles past my turnoff to Spokane and was, indeed, headed straight for Carson City. The reason that scenery looked so darned beautiful and fresh and new and unseen was because, well, it *was* beautiful and fresh, but more important, it was also completely *new* and most assuredly *unseen*. Just in case you were wondering, it was just as beautiful and fresh, though markedly less *novel* as I traversed the ninety miles back to the turnoff to Spokane.

A SLICE OF INSIGHT:
HERE AND THERE

The key, I learned from this rather lengthy but visually appealing drive, is that you have to be mind*ful*, not mind*less*, in your quest to truly be present in the here and now. If you're not on the right path to reach the destination you want, you certainly *can* enjoy the *moment*, it's just that you might enjoy it in a *radically* different *location* and on a *markedly* different *time line* than you initially planned. So it goes, that sometimes even our very best intentions can lead us astray, and our most powerful convictions can be misleading when we allow ourselves to be in the right *moment* in the wrong *manner*.

What does it look like to practice mindfulness *thoughtfully*? Good question. One I wish I had asked ten or fifteen (rather than

> **S**ometimes even our very best intentions can lead us astray, and our most powerful convictions can be misleading when we allow ourselves to be in the right *moment* in the wrong *manner*.

ninety) extra miles into my drive. Upon reflection, though, I believe it's about being aware *of*, and fully present *in*, your "this-moment" experience in a way that enhances the "big vision" for your life. It's about looking at the "you are here" marker on the map of your life, and recognizing and appreciating what's good and wonderful about right now. And it's about keeping an eye on your destination—the "there" you're traveling to, with full awareness of why it's special, too. It's about staying alert during your journey, not just sleepwalking or daydreaming or joyriding through it. It's about knowing when to be focused on a specific outcome (your destination) but also about knowing how to navigate where you are right now, and feeling confident that detours and scenic routes can *add* to your trip

> **M**indfulness is a conscious choice to be simultaneously present in this moment, in your life, and in your eager but relaxed anticipation for what is to come.

rather than *detract* from it. And, it's about using the tools at your disposal to provide information or insight when you want it or need it (including, but not limited to, highway signs and road maps in my case).

Mindfulness is a conscious choice to be simultaneously present in this moment, in your life, and in your eager but relaxed anticipation for what is to come. That way, no matter where you've been, where you are now, or where you end up, you can see the exquisite beauty at every stage of your journey. Even when the journey is a little longer or a bit more out of the way than you anticipated!

MINDFULNESS BITE BY BITE: KNOWING YOUR NOW AND LOOKING FORWARD TO LATER

1. Think about times in your life when you were in the *right* moment in the *wrong* way. What were the *consequences* you experienced, and how did you *feel* as a result?

2. Think about times in your life when you have been present in *this moment*, in *your life*, and in your eager but relaxed anticipation for *what is to come*? How did you *feel* during those instances, and what kind of *results* did they produce for you?

3. What practices can you put into place (or eliminate) that will help maximize your tendency toward *mindfulness* and *meaning* both *now* and *later*?

The Best (and the Worst) of Zen-tentions

It had been one of those weeks followed by one of those week-ends. A crazy schedule, crummy weather, clingy kids—the tenseness trifecta. Instead of drinking excessively or submerging myself in several pints of Häagen-Dazs (though I considered both), I threw myself into a homemaker frenzy of epic proportions. Somehow, amid the temper tantrums (which deftly alternated between my children and myself) I had managed to clean the produce drawers in the fridge (*most* of which should have been classified as science experiments) and pay the massive stack of bills (*all* of which were late, requiring me to hand-write "thank you" with a little smiley face on the memo line of each check). The only thing that kept me bordering on sanity (I decline to confess which side of the border I was on) was the promise of one glorious hour of silence, mindfulness, and me-time. Yoga class. It couldn't come soon enough.

I struggled to the door, my eighteen-month-old clinging to my leg like one of those Velcro koalas that hug the end of your pencil. I pried him loose, gently transferred him to my husband (as gentle as you can be with a doe-eyed wild animal of a mama's boy), and said, "G'day, mate." I gunned it out of the driveway and briefly wondered what my family would do if I simply just kept driving. But I knew that after a luxurious hour of silence I would feel differently. I would gently enter "the zone," reunite breath and body as one, and would then be drawn home again to inhale the scent of freshly bathed, pajama-clad children ready to engage in the evening cuddle postures. Yes, I would return. But for now, all I could imagine were their little hands giving me the thumbs-up and their faces cheering me on, shouting, "Bring on the pranayama, Mama!"

I sighed, turned on the satellite radio to the "spa channel," where I was thrilled to hear my favorite yoga chant melting its way through my speakers. I turned it up like a favorite rock anthem and thought, "Right on! This will totally jump-start my Zen." In my frenetic state, I figured that since I was running late for class, if I listened to the chant on the way, I'd gradually transition myself into a trancelike state precisely upon my arrival at the studio. What luck! And then the luck began to slowly drain from my evening, just as the color drained from my face as I recognized the red and blue lights flashing in my rearview mirror.

I pulled over to the side of the highway and waited for the officer. He sauntered slowly up to the car (maybe he was listening to the spa channel, too?) and said, "Ma'am, I pulled you over for speeding. You were going sixty in a fifty. Where are you headed in such a hurry?" "Uh, well, honestly? To yoga class," I offered, albeit a bit sheepishly. "I see. Doesn't seem to make much sense, does it, ma'am?" "No," I halfheartedly agreed, "I guess not." "May I see your driver's license, proof of insurance, and your registration please?" "Sure," I stammered, "I've got them right here." I started digging through my purse, which held approximately six weeks' worth of receipts that tightly encased my driver's license like an Egyptian mummy, only without the cache of priceless artifacts (unless you call four petrified gummy bears and a lone McDonald's french fry priceless artifacts). He was already getting a bit perturbed when I had to pause to scrape the dried-on bit of berry smoothie off the corner of the picture before I handed it to him. "Hope you're not going to check the weight," I joked with a nervous laugh. He didn't laugh back.

He lifted the license up to the light and said, "Is this your current address, Ms. Davis?" My stomach turned. "Oh, uh, well, actually, um, no, it's not. We, um, built a new home on the prairie back there and, uh, I haven't had time to change the address yet." "And did you move recently?" He asked. "Well, uh, recently . . . it . . . as a matter of fact . . . it was, oh, let's see, uh . . . hmmm, I guess it's been eighteen months now. Wow, how time flies!" I offered, with that high-pitched, incredulous, completely unbelievable lilt. "But I had a baby right after we moved in and, well, I kind of lost track of time. You know how it goes." (Tense giggle.) He tilted his head and raised his left eyebrow. "No, ma'am, I don't."

Suddenly he morphed into my father and I could have sworn that he asked me if I had been the one who dumped the entire bag of sugar on the kitchen floor and then made sand art with it. "Ma'am, did you know you're supposed to change your address within one month of moving, otherwise it's a hundred-dollar fine?" "*Wow*, oh boy, no. No, I certainly did *not* know that. But . . . I guess I do now. I'll take care of that right away. I mean tomorrow, of course. When they're open. Because they're obviously not open now." (Attempted endearing half smile, which contorted into edgy lip purse with matching eye twitch.)

"Okay, can I see your registration, please?" "Oh, yes. Let me get that for you." I opened the glove box, and out cascaded the receipt for every oil change I've ever gotten, a bottle of dried-out hand sanitizer, a stray mitten, extra napkins and straws from just about every restaurant in my hometown, a lavender aromatherapy disk, maps for cities I don't think I've ever actually visited, approximately fourteen CDs, a wadded-up diaper, and three distinct flavors of lip balm, none of which I care for. But no registration. "He, he, he. My mobile command center needs a better commander, I think." He raised his other eyebrow. Silence. (Soft chuckle that faded off into a nervous gulp.)

I dug through the side pockets of the doors and finally found the registration in the console between the seats. "Whew, I knew I had it here somewhere!" He looked at the registration. "Ms. Davis, did you realize that your registration isn't signed? And did you also know that that's another fine?" "Um, I guess I didn't even know you were supposed to sign it. Well, I guess it's true you learn something new every single day of your life, isn't it? I'm just racking them up today!" (Unconvincing and a bit disturbing half giggle/half warble.)

I was starting to shake now. This experience was sucking the Zen right out of the car. I could see it delicately spiraling up and out of the window as I looked up at the officer. I think it spelled out the word "namaste" in the tradition of skywriting. I glanced at the clock, which I imagined was a time bomb relentlessly ticking its way toward destroying what once was a fabulous hour of self-care. Then the ticking morphed into the tapping of calculator keys totaling up the biggest citation ever written for a minor traffic infraction.

"Now all I need is your insurance card." "Oh, yes," I said, fully flustered by this point. "Let me see here." I pulled out the insurance card. For my previous insurance carrier. Whom I had transferred my policy from well over nine months earlier. "Oops," I said, lifting my shoulders and eyebrows in a show of painful recognition, "wrong carrier. But wait! I know I have the new one here somewhere, because I remember he faxed it to me." I lifted the bin of papers from the backseat and sifted through it until I finally stumbled on the crumpled piece of paper. "Whew!" I said. "That was close." I could see my hands shaking as I handed it to him.

"Ma'am, did you know that your insurance card is expired?" he asked, now hovering somewhere between annoyance and outright disgust. "And that that's *another* fine of nearly four hundred dollars?" I wanted to bellow at the top of my lungs, "Do you think you could start a sentence with anything other than '*Ma'am, did you know?*' Because don't you think that if I *knew* I wouldn't be here and would instead be perfecting my Downward-Facing *Dog* as opposed to bearing witness to my Downward-Spiraling *Psyche* with matching Downward-Dwindling Bank Account courtesy of the many, many, many traffic fines I'm racking up as we speak?" Instead I gingerly offered, "Wow, uh, I gotta say, *huh*. No, no, no, uh, *no*, I did *not* realize that." (Quasi-psychotic snickering ensued.)

"Wait here, please," he said, shaking his head as he walked back toward his cruiser to call it in. I glanced first at the clock, grieving my lost hour of bliss, and then up at the rearview mirror. And then it started. At the precise moment that the flow series started in yoga class, I was commencing my own personal flow series. I saw the first tear gently wind its way down the side of my face. I looked straight up, trying to stave it off until he handed over the world's biggest ticket, but it was no use. The next tear followed suit, and then another, and then another. And the floodgates flew open. I started weeping openly, uncontrollably, almost bordering on "the ugly cry." My shoulders hunched over and I sobbed and sobbed and sobbed as he sauntered back to the car and handed me my documents.

And there I went. "I'm so sorry, Officer. I'm a really safe driver, really. I've just had this really crappy weekend and my kids were so needy and all my bills were late and the cucumbers were all penicillin-y and I'm so tired and all I wanted was to just go to yoga for one hour to try to let go of it and I'm just so sorry because I never speed and I didn't even know I had to change the address and I had my old car insurance for twenty years and so this company is totally new to me and I sign so many things I can't believe I didn't sign the registration and I'm just really, really having a bad day and my pranayama is gone, gone, gone." (Massive snort, followed by disturbing gurgle, followed by quivering sigh.)

He looked at me with what at that moment I read as compassion, but what I later interpreted as sheer terror and said, "I'm going to let you off with a warning this time. But slow it down. And sign your registration. And change your address. And get your new insurance card. And enjoy your yoga class." And he walked away. I took a deep breath and realized that, in that moment of profound gratitude for his leniency (and for not calling the mental health hotline to have me carted away), I was actually *in* the moment. Mind and body as one. Fully present. My Zen wound its way back into the car. I felt peaceful again.

And then I realized that, throughout this whole interchange, my radio had been blaring that yoga mantra song at about forty decibels, making the haunting, rhythmic melody the perfect (actually, perfectly hilarious) sound track to this ridiculous ordeal. And my tears turned to laughter as I shook my head and drove back home, hugging the speed limit as closely as I hugged my kids that night. I guess if nothing else, I've always got the best of Zen-tentions. That has to count for something, right?

A SLICE OF INSIGHT: ESCAPE TO ENGAGEMENT

Ah, the paradoxes that poise us for growth. As I look back at that whole incident, it makes me laugh to this day—not only because I've never since been able to look my neighbor, a sheriff, in the eye, knowing that he heard the entire tale of the "crazy yoga lady" over his radio that night and in report the next morning. Certainly, that would be enough to make me continue to laugh but there's more. I'm still totally flabbergasted that the whole manner in which I tried to make it to yoga that night was in stark contradiction to the *true* practice of mindfulness. I was in such a frenetic, stressed-out state that I felt I had to *escape* from life in order to *engage* in it. Ridiculous? Yes. Uncommon? I don't think so. The whole point is that you don't have to *go* somewhere special or *do* something specific to be mindful.

> You don't have to *go* somewhere special or *do* something specific to be mindful. On the contrary, all you have to do is *be* in the moment and experience all it has to offer.

On the contrary, all you have to do is *be* in the moment and experience all it has to offer.

I had so many opportunities that night to get back in to my "moment-ous" state of mind. And yet, even as I got closer to a "practice" of mindfulness (yoga class), I wasn't actually "practicing" mindfulness (being truly present in all of my experiences, good or bad, stressful or blissful). That's an important distinction: There is a difference between a "practice" of mindfulness (like yoga and meditation) and the process of "practicing" mindfulness, which involves being present in the moment regardless of what you're doing *and* being nonjudgmental of both yourself and the situation. I *wasn't* present in my departure from home (thus, the need to pry Velcro boy from my fast-paced stride as I left). I *wasn't* present on the drive (thus, the speeding stop). I *wasn't* present to the fact that this whole incident was a clear example of the disarray in my schedule, my car, and my life (thus, the ever-growing total of the potential citation). And I *wasn't* even present to the yoga chant blaring from my speakers as I sobbed uncontrollably to the taken-aback officer.

> There is a difference between a "practice" of mindfulness (like yoga and meditation) and the process of "practicing" mindfulness, which involves being present in the moment regardless of what you're doing *and* being nonjudgmental of both yourself and the situation.

But after all was said and done, I returned home, exhausted but engaged, and I *was* exceptionally present to my children, husband, and home, grateful to be reminded of what it feels like to truly be *in that moment and in my life*. And that was a far better lesson than I could have learned in yoga class any day.

After all, I think we sometimes mistakenly assume that we need to gain our wisdom and grow our skills from a teacher or a textbook in a classroom or a conference, when often the very best learning and the most profound transformations are produced when we see *ourselves* as the educators, each *moment* as our mentor, and our *lives* as the learning environment. I'm pretty convinced that's a far better way to jump-start your Zen and create a "moment-ous" life than any other approach I can think of. But who wants to think of any other approaches when this one seems to work so well?

MINDFULNESS BITE BY BITE: THE PRACTICE OF PRACTICING

1. Are there times in your life when you have thought you needed to *escape* from life in order to *engage* in it? What results did that produce for you?

2. What ideas do you have for designing a truly "moment-ous" experience each day of your life? How can you begin embracing each moment *today*?

3. In the future, how might you make it a *practice* to commit to *practicing* mindfulness in everyday tasks, whether you are scrubbing sinks or sharing a meal, solving world crises or carpooling the kids?

AFTERWORD

So the end, as they say, is actually the beginning. Throughout this book you have explored the merits of perspective, connection, adaptability, resilience, and release, as well as an array of strategies for integrating those principles and their related practices into your life. You've had the opportunity to honor the role that both laughter and tears play in creating a meaningful life experience, in celebratory moments and in challenging times. With all good fortune, you have delighted in those messages along with a few exquisite slices of pie. I trust that as you read, you committed to develop a personal path to *live mindfully* rather than to *act mindlessly* each day of your life, regardless of your circumstances. Every human being deserves the opportunity to enjoy the "moment-ous" process of living with joy and intention. And, it is my sincere hope (and strong recommendation) that from this day forward you will consistently look for and savor every opportunity you can to laugh, cry, and eat some pie. Bon voyage, and bon appétit!

Deanna Davis, PhD, is the author of *Laugh, Cry, Eat Some Pie, Living with Intention*, and *The Law of Attraction in Action*. She is a professional speaker and entertainer, and the creator of the one-woman-show *Womanhood: The Divine Comedy*.

Known for her characteristic blend of humor and how-to, Deanna's speaking and writing focuses on living life by design, rather than by default, and on creating extraordinary success and satisfaction on your own terms. She integrates cutting-edge research from the disciplines of Positive Psychology, mind/body health, neuroscience, and leadership with practical strategies for creating change.

Deanna teaches personal and professional success strategies based on "the big power of small," since small changes, small steps, and small investments lead to big—and lasting—results over time. By taking small steps, you can harness the momentum from minor wins to help you sail to your next level of success and satisfaction. By using incremental changes to detour around the fear and stress that can undermine your best intentions, you learn to use your internal compass to travel from where you are now to where you want to be.

Deanna is an admitted laughaholic and a strong proponent

of adding chocolate as a key component of the USDA Food Pyramid.

Visit Deanna online at www.deannadavis.net, where you will find free resources to help you create your ideal life on your own terms starting today. On the website you can also learn more about her events, products, and speaking services.